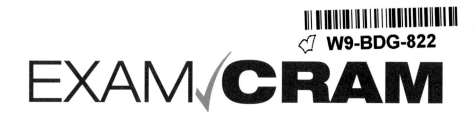

✓ W9-BDG-822

Nursing Assistant Certification Examination Cram Sheet

This cram sheet provides a quick reference of the facts and figures you need for Testing Now Tips (TNTs) as you enter the testing center to complete your certification examination process. Use these TNTs to make notes on a sheet of scrap paper while in the testing center. Review the glossary as a last-minute cram strategy before entering the testing center. Good luck.

- ▶ Get a good night's sleep.
- ▶ Do not work the night before the examination.
- ▶ Avoid alcohol or excessive caffeine before the examination.
- ▶ Take your time with the test questions, but pace yourself to finish the examination within the allotted time.
- ▶ Read each question thoroughly and completely before selecting the best answer.
- ▶ Do not panic if you are not familiar with a question.
- ▶ Believe in yourself; we do! You can succeed!

IMPORTANT HEALTH-CARE LAWS TO REMEMBER

HIPAA: Health Insurance Portability and Accountability Act (1966):
Law requiring health information about resident be kept confidential except as authorized by the resident.

OBRA: Omnibus Budget Reconciliation Act:
Federal act that addresses the safety, welfare, and happiness of patients. The act also addresses the quality of training and continuing education of nursing assistants.

PSDA: Patient Self-Determination Act:
Federal law that protects the resident's right to accept or refuse medical or surgical care and treatment, including the right to prepare written guidelines (advance directive) outlining instructions in such matters in the event the resident cannot represent self.

INDIRECT CARE REMINDERS

▶ Wash your hands before and after each procedure and between care for each resident.

▶ Greet each resident by name and introduce yourself.

▶ Before beginning and throughout, explain the procedure to the resident.

▶ Provide privacy for the resident.

▶ Close the door or curtain.

▶ Promote and ensure resident rights.

▶ Use standard precautions where applicable.

▶ Promote resident comfort and safety.

▶ Report/record all procedures, results, and resident's response to care

▶ Clean, replenish, and store supplies and equipment.

REMEMBER THE RACE SYSTEM FOR FIRE SAFETY

Remove residents who are in immediate danger.

Activate the alarm to alert others.

Contain the fire by closing doors.

Extinguish the fire or **E**vacuate if instructed to do so.

MEDICAL ABBREVIATIONS

Abd.: Abdomen
ADLs: Activities of daily living
ax: Axillary; under the arm
B/P: Blood pressure
BS: Blood sugar
BSC: Bedside commode
C & S: Culture and sensitivity
CVA: Cerebrovascular accident, stroke
DNR: Do not resuscitate
AMI: Acute Myocardial Infarct
Ht.: Height
I.V.: Intravenous
mL: Milliliter
MRSA: Methicillin-Resistant Staphylococcus Aureus
I & O: Intake and output
N & V: Nausea and vomiting
N.P.O.: Nothing by mouth
02: Oxygen
P.O.: By mouth
PRN: Whenever necessary
R.O.M.: Range of motion
STAT: Immediately; at once
STD/STI: Sexually transmitted disease; sexually transmitted illness
TM: Tympanic membrane
TPR: Temperature, pulse, and respirations
VS: Vital signs
Rx: Treatment
w-c: Wheelchair
Wt.: Weight
WNL: Within normal limits
XR: X-ray

MEASUREMENTS

1 teaspoon equals 5 cc (or 5 mL)
1 ounce (oz.) equals 30 cc (or mL)
1 cup (8 oz.) equals 240 cc (or mL)

VITAL SIGNS

Average temperature: 98.6
Average pulse (Adults): 60–100
Average respiration (Adults): 12–20
Average blood pressure (Adults): 120/80

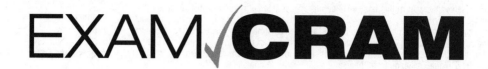

CNA
Certified Nursing Assistant
Second Edition

Linda Whitenton, Marty Walker

Pearson
800 East 96th Street
Indianapolis, Indiana 46240 USA

9/17

CNA Certified Nursing Assistant Exam Cram, Second Edition

ISBN-13: 978-0-7897-5886-6

ISBN-10: 0-7897-5886-5

Library of Congress Control Number: 2017938512

Printed in the United States of America

1   17

Trademarks

All terms mentioned in this book that are known to be trademarks or service marks have been appropriately capitalized. Pearson IT Certification cannot attest to the accuracy of this information. Use of a term in this book should not be regarded as affecting the validity of any trademark or service mark.

Warning and Disclaimer

Every effort has been made to make this book as complete and as accurate as possible, but no warranty or fitness is implied. The information provided is on an "as is" basis. The authors and the publisher shall have neither liability nor responsibility to any person or entity with respect to any loss or damages arising from the information contained in this book.

Special Sales

For information about buying this title in bulk quantities, or for special sales opportunities (which may include electronic versions; custom cover designs; and content particular to your business, training goals, marketing focus, or branding interests), please contact our corporate sales department at corpsales@pearsoned.com or (800) 382-3419.

For government sales inquiries, please contact governmentsales@pearsoned.com.

For questions about sales outside the U.S., please contact intlcs@pearson.com.

Editor-in-Chief
Mark Taub

Product Line Manager
Brett Bartow

Acquisitions Editor
Michelle Newcomb

Development Editor
Christopher Cleveland

Managing Editor
Sandra Schroeder

Senior Project Editor
Tonya Simpson

Copy Editor
Barbara Hacha

Indexer
Cheryl Lenser

Proofreader
Sasirekha Durairajan

Technical Editor
Steve Picray

Publishing Coordinator
Vanessa Evans

Cover Designer
Chuti Prasertsith

Compositor
codeMantra

Contents at a Glance

Contents

About the Authors

Marty Walker has practiced nursing for the past 39 years at the vocational nursing level as a registered nurse, and at the master's level. Marty began her nursing career as a licensed practical nurse, receiving her vocational education certificate from Atlantic Vocational School in Pompano Beach, Florida, in 1979. In 1982, she earned the associate degree in nursing from Broward Community College in Davie, Florida. She worked for more than 10 years as a staff nurse in telemetry, critical care, and emergency nursing before completing a bachelor of science degree in nursing from Florida International University in Miami, Florida. In 1995, she began teaching medical-surgical nursing at Ivy Tech State College in Sellersburg, Indiana.

After relocating to Miami, Marty accepted a position as Nurse Clinical Educator for three cardiac units at Jackson Memorial Hospital. She attained a Master's in Nursing Science in Nursing Education from Barry University in Miami Shores, Florida, in 2003. Marty's love of teaching led her to Mercy Hospital's School of Practical Nursing, along with adjunct teaching positions at Florida International University and Barry University. In Miami, Marty added pediatrics to her teaching expertise. She taught medical-surgical nursing for a short time at Pensacola State College in Pensacola, Florida, before accepting a full-time associate professor position at Northwest Florida State College, where she taught in the RN-BSN program as well as the associate degree nursing program. She is now the director for both programs. Marty's expertise also includes test construction. She has led the faculty at NWF State College in improving the success rates of students enrolled in the program as well as their success on the NCLEX-RN. Marty's versatility extends to her clinical practice as she completed the family nurse practitioner certificate program at the University of South Alabama in Mobile, Alabama, where she also completed her Doctorate in Nursing Practice in 2014. Marty has volunteered as the director of nursing services, as a nurse practitioner, and as board president for the Crossroads Medical Center Clinic in Valparaiso, Florida, since 2007.

Linda Whitenton began a 45-year nursing career in 1967 as a nursing assistant in Paducah, Kentucky. Following her graduation from Murray State University's BSN program in 1970, she practiced in mental health, pediatrics, and medical-surgical nursing. Teaching nursing assistants, emergency medical technicians, and unit secretaries in a Mississippi hospital cemented her love for teaching in her role as a hospital in-service education director in the early 1970s. She accepted her first teaching position at Northeast Mississippi Community College in 1975. While at NEMC, she taught fundamentals, medical-surgical nursing, management, and psychiatric nursing and served as assistant director and director of the program for seven years. In 1977, Linda earned her master's of science degree in nursing at the Mississippi University for Women, which also afforded her the family nurse clinician credential. In 1987, she relocated to Florida and accepted a position as associate director of nursing for the associate degree nursing program at St. Petersburg College in St. Petersburg.

While at SPC, she designed curriculum for more than 1,000 employees of the Pinellas County EMS, taught LPN transitional students at night, and practiced part time at the Bayfront Medical Center Trauma Center.

During her 35 years of teaching, Linda continued to practice in emergency nursing, urological nursing, and as a nurse clinician. Linda also earned 30 hours of post-masters work in anthropology and educational psychology. In 2004, she returned to clinical practice as the director of nursing/vice president for a Mississippi community hospital. While there, she received a national award for outstanding nursing leadership. She returned to Florida in 2000 to design and direct a new AD nursing program for Northwest Florida State College, formerly Okaloosa-Walton College, the first of seven health programs now in place at the college. Linda served as associate dean of Health Technology for three years, adding administrative oversight for the health programs she launched during her eight-year tenure at NWFSC. In 2008, she retired from the college, receiving the honor of Emeritus Associate Dean and Director of Nursing. In 2015, Linda accepted an interim position as campus dean at Pensacola State College, where she now serves as director of Nursing and Emergency Medical Services, overseeing the nursing programs, the emergency medical service programs, the surgical technology, and the newly designed patient care technician program. Linda has worked with Rinehart and Associates Nursing Review, a nurse-owned company that offers review courses for graduates preparing for their examination to become licensed RNs or LPNs. Linda is a Certified Nurse Educator, CNE, and a member of Sigma Theta Tau International Nursing Society.

About the Technical Editor

Steven M. Picray is a medical surgical registered nurse in a major metropolitan hospital. He has also been a Baptist pastor and a computer programmer. He has a bachelor's and a master's degrees in theology, a B.S.N., and is currently pursuing his master's degree in nursing to become a nurse practitioner.

Dedication

*We dedicate this book to the compassionate and caring nursing
assistants everywhere, who dedicate their lives
to caring for our precious elders.*

Acknowledgments

We wish to thank Kathy McNair for her superlative technical assistance, her encouragement, caring, and expertise in all she does for nursing education.

A special thanks goes to Mrs. Jeanece C. Ridge, former instructor, Nursing Assistant Program and current instructor, Practical Nursing Program at Okaloosa Technical College in Fort Walton Beach, Florida, for her thorough review of our first edition.

We also thank our families for their love and patience.

Contact the Nursing Board in Your Area

Because nursing standards sometimes vary by state due to differing legal concerns at the state level, you should check the Nurse Aid Registries at National Council of State Boards of Nursing website for your area at https://www.ncsbn.org/725.htm.

Companion Website

Register this book to get access to the Pearson Test Prep practice test software and other study materials plus additional bonus content. Check this site regularly for new and updated postings written by the author that provide further insight into the more troublesome topics on the exam. Be sure to check the box that you would like to hear from us to receive updates and exclusive discounts on future editions of this product or related products.

To access this companion website, follow these steps:

1. Go to www.pearsonITcertification.com/register and log in or create a new account.

2. Enter the ISBN: 9780789758866.

3. Answer the challenge question as proof of purchase.

4. Click the **Access Bonus Content** link in the Registered Products section of your account page to be taken to the page where your downloadable content is available.

Please note that many of our companion content files can be very large, especially image and video files.

If you are unable to locate the files for this title by following the preceding steps, visit www.pearsonITcertification.com/contact and select the "Site Problems/ Comments" option. Our customer service representatives will assist you.

Pearson Test Prep Practice Test Software

As noted previously, this book comes complete with the Pearson Test Prep practice test software containing three full exams. These practice tests are available to you either online or as an offline Windows application. To access the practice exams that were developed with this book, please see the instructions in the card inserted in the sleeve in the back of the book. This card includes a unique access code that enables you to activate your exams in the Pearson Test Prep software.

Accessing the Pearson Test Prep Software Online

The online version of this software can be used on any device with a browser and connectivity to the Internet, including desktop machines, tablets, and smartphones. To start using your practice exams online, follow these steps:

1. Go to http://www.PearsonTestPrep.com.

2. Select **Pearson IT Certification** as your product group.

3. Enter your email/password for your account. If you don't have an account on PearsonITCertification.com or CiscoPress.com, you will need to establish one by going to PearsonITCertification.com/join.

4. In the My Products tab, click the **Activate New Product** button.

5. Enter the access code printed on the insert card in the back of your book to activate your product.

6. The product will now be listed in your My Products page. Click the **Exams** button to launch the exam settings screen and start your exam.

Accessing the Pearson Test Prep Software Offline

If you want to study offline, you can download and install the Windows version of the Pearson Test Prep software. There is a download link for this software on the book's companion website, or you can enter this link in your browser:

http://www.pearsonitcertification.com/content/downloads/pcpt/engine.zip

To access the book's companion website and the software, follow these steps:

1. Register your book by going to: PearsonITCertification.com/register and entering the ISBN: 9780789758866.

2. Respond to the challenge questions.

3. Go to your account page and select the **Registered Products** tab.

4. Click the **Access Bonus Content** link under the product listing.

5. Click the **Install Pearson Test Prep Desktop Version** link under the Practice Exams section of the page to download the software.

6. After the software finishes downloading, unzip all the files on your computer.

7. Double-click the application file to start the installation, and follow the onscreen instructions to complete the registration.

8. After the installation is complete, launch the application and select **Activate Exam** button on the My Products tab.

9. Click the **Activate a Product** button in the Activate Product Wizard.

10. Enter the unique access code found on the card in the sleeve in the back of your book, and click the **Activate** button.

11. Click **Next** and then the **Finish** button to download the exam data to your application.

12. You can now start using the practice exams by selecting the product and clicking the **Open Exam** button to open the exam settings screen.

Note that the offline and online versions will synch together, so saved exams and grade results recorded on one version will be available to you on the other as well.

Customizing Your Exams

When you are in the exam settings screen, you can choose to take exams in one of three modes:

- ▶ Study Mode
- ▶ Practice Exam Mode
- ▶ Flash Card Mode

Study Mode enables you to fully customize your exams and review answers as you are taking the exam. This is typically the mode you would use first to assess your knowledge and identify information gaps. Practice Exam Mode locks certain customization options because it is presenting a realistic exam experience. Use this mode when you are preparing to test your exam readiness. Flash Card Mode strips out the answers and presents you with only the question stem. This mode is great for late stage preparation when you want to challenge yourself to provide answers without the benefit of seeing multiple choice options. This mode will not provide the detailed score reports that the other two modes will, so it should not be used if you are trying to identify knowledge gaps.

In addition to these three modes, you will be able to select the source of your questions. You can choose to take exams that cover all the chapters, or you can narrow your selection to a single chapter or the chapters that make up specific parts in the book. All chapters are selected by default. If you want to narrow your focus to individual chapters, deselect all the chapters, and then select only those on which you wish to focus in the Objectives area.

You can also select the exam banks on which to focus. Each exam bank comes complete with a full exam of questions that cover topics in every chapter. The three exams printed in the book are also available online. You can have the test engine serve up exams from all three banks or just from one individual bank by selecting the desired banks in the exam bank area.

You can make several other customizations to your exam from the exam settings screen, such as the time of the exam, the number of questions served up, whether to randomize questions and answers, whether to show the number of correct answers for multiple answer questions, or whether to serve up only specific types of questions. You can also create custom test banks by selecting only questions that you have marked or questions on which you have added notes.

Updating Your Exams

If you are using the online version of the Pearson Test Prep software, you should always have access to the latest version of the software as well as the exam data. If you are using the Windows desktop version, every time you launch the software, it will check to see if there are any updates to your exam data and automatically download any changes that were made since the last time you used the software. This requires that you are connected to the Internet at the time you launch the software.

Sometimes, due to many factors, the exam data may not fully download when you activate your exam. If you find that figures or exhibits are missing, you may need to manually update your exams.

To update a particular exam you have already activated and downloaded, select the **Tools** tab and select the **Update Products** button. Again, this is an issue only with the desktop Windows application.

If you want to check for updates to the Pearson Test Prep exam engine software, Windows desktop version, simply select the **Tools** tab and select the **Update Application** button. This will ensure you are running the latest version of the software engine.

We Want to Hear from You!

As the reader of this book, *you* are our most important critic and commentator. We value your opinion and want to know what we're doing right, what we could do better, what areas you'd like to see us publish in, and any other words of wisdom you're willing to pass our way.

We welcome your comments. You can email or write to let us know what you did or didn't like about this book—as well as what we can do to make our books better.

Please note that we cannot help you with technical problems related to the topic of this book.

When you write, please be sure to include this book's title and author as well as your name and email address. We will carefully review your comments and share them with the author and editors who worked on the book.

Email: feedback@pearsonitcertification.com

Mail: Pearson IT Certification
         ATTN: Reader Feedback
         800 East 96th Street
         Indianapolis, IN 46240 USA

Reader Services

Register your copy of *CNA Certified Nursing Assistant Exam Cram* at www.pearsonitcertification.com for convenient access to downloads, updates, and corrections as they become available. To start the registration process, go to www.pearsonitcertification.com/register and log in or create an account*. Enter the product ISBN 9780789758866 and click Submit. When the process is complete, you will find any available bonus content under Registered Products.

*Be sure to check the box that you would like to hear from us to receive exclusive discounts on future editions of this product.

CHAPTER ONE

What You Need to Know to Prepare for the Exam

The Certified Nursing Assistant Examination, referred to as the *exam*, consists of both a written examination (the WE) and the clinical skills test (the CST).

The written (oral) examination content outline, effective 2016, also known as the National Nurse Aide Assessment Program (NNAAP), is published by the National Council of State Boards of Nursing (NCSBN). The examination content is based on a national survey of the most important findings of the components of nurse aide practice (Table 1.1). The content and its weight on the examination follows:

TABLE 1.1   The 2016 National Nurse Aide Assessment Program (NNAAP) Written (Oral) Examination Content Outline

Content Domain	Weighting of Content Domain	Key Knowledge Focus
I. Physical Care Skills	14%	
A. Activities of Daily Living		
1. Hygiene		Handwashing; Risk Factors
2. Dressing and Grooming		Dehydration; Dietary
3. Nutrition and Hydration		Restrictions; Feeding Complications
4. Elimination		
5. Rest/Sleep/Comfort		Incontinence Care
		Reporting Pain
B. Basic Nursing Skills	39%	
1. Infection Control		Spread of Infection;
2. Safety/Emergency		Airborne Precautions; Biohazards Disposal; PPE
3. Therapeutic and Technical Procedures		Call System; High Risk, Injury; Fire
4. Data Collection and Reporting		
		Disaster Procedure
C. Restorative Skills	8%	BLS; Airway Obstruction
1. Prevention		Ambulation; Safety
2. Self-care/Independence		Safety Alarms

Content Domain	Weighting of Content Domain	Key Knowledge Focus
II. Psychosocial Care Skills		
A. Emotional and Mental Health Needs	11%	Loneliness; Isolation
B. Spiritual and Cultural Needs	2%	Signs of Suicide Ideation
III. Role of the Nurse Aide		
A. Communication	8%	Client Plan of Care
B. Client Rights	7%	Client Identification
C. Legal and Ethical Behavior	3%	HIPPA
D. Member of the Health Care Team	8%	Dignity
		Privacy Confidentiality
		Reporting
		Workplace Activities
Total	100%	

Note: A cross-reference table in Appendix A will further assist you in concentrating on content and key knowledge review.

Source: National Council of State Boards of Nursing. (2016). www.ncsbn.org

You must successfully pass both the WE and the CST to pass the certification examination. Specific details on both the WE and the CST, as well as tips on preparing for each portion, follow.

Taking the Written Examination

The written examination (WE) is a computerized exam with a time limit, usually two hours. Test sites are regional or local, depending on the state jurisdiction. We recommend you follow the instructions given by the testing center without exception and arrive at least 30 minutes early or, if you're traveling a long distance, arrive a day early to locate the testing center and the most judicious travel route to avoid delays. Two forms of identification are required:

▶ A current, unexpired driver's license, state-issued identification card or military ID card, one of which is a picture ID. You must also present a current photo along with your readable signature. You should present a name that exactly matches your name as listed on your Admission-To-Test (ATT) letter.

▶ The second form of identification must also have your signature on it. Examples of second forms of identification include credit cards and Social Security cards. The card must also have your signature, signed prior to testing day. If any signs of alteration or damage to the card are suspected, you may be denied admittance to test.

Dress warmly but do not bring anything to the testing area. Leave all personal items (purses, cell phones, calculators, and so on) outside the testing areas. You will be issued testing materials as needed. Other helpful tips for a successful testing experience are as follows:

▶ Get a good night's sleep.

▶ Don't work the night before the examination.

▶ Avoid alcohol or excessive caffeine before the examination.

▶ Eat a light but well-balanced meal (protein, carbohydrates, and fats plus liquids) while studying and before the exam. You (and your brain) need energy and maximum recall to be well prepared! Although heavy sugars give you an energy boost, avoid them because you might experience a sudden dip in blood sugar, causing fatigue and nausea. You might also become hungry later when you cannot eat, for example, when taking the exam. To avoid sudden dips in blood sugar bring protein snacks, such as dry roasted nuts or cheese crackers.

▶ Take your time with the test questions, but pace yourself to finish the examination within the allotted time.

▶ Read each question thoroughly and completely before selecting the best answer.

▶ Don't panic if you are not familiar with a question. Remember the Testing Now Tips (TNTs) on your Cram Sheet.

▶ Believe in yourself; we do! You can succeed!

Passing scores for the WE vary from state to state. Expect to earn at least a 70% for a passing score. You might have to wait two to three days for results. If needed, follow directions for scheduling a repeat the examination.

To successfully pass the Critical Skills Test (CST), you must earn a score of at least 70% while following each critical step with 100% accuracy. You should be given the opportunity to correct any missed checkpoints or other aspects of the skill during your performance; however, when you have finished a particular skill and progress to the next one, you will not be able to correct a mistake made on the previous one. If you need to repeat any portion of the CST, you'll receive directions from the evaluator regarding subsequent testing opportunities according to each state's testing guidelines.

Some helpful tips for success on the CST are as follows:

▶ Practice, practice, practice!

▶ Follow each skill/procedure exactly as you learned them in your nurse aide program; this is *not* the time to improvise or take shortcuts!

▶ Follow safety standards and include them in your skill performance. This includes, but is not limited to, handwashing, handling of soiled items, and other safety precautions. These are examples of indirect care standards that will be evaluated with each skill. For example, *prior* to performing a skill, you must actually use water and wash your hands; the evaluator will tell you after you've washed your hands correctly for the first time that you can tell him or her when you would wash your hands rather than actually washing them for each subsequent skill.

▶ Work confidently and efficiently; you must complete each procedure in a timely manner.

▶ Remember, the skills test is designed to measure *your* competency; you will not be given assistance by the evaluator except to remind you of time limitations related to the skill performance.

▶ Imagine getting the good news: You passed! Imagery is a powerful tool to encourage success.

Find a quiet location each day where you can concentrate and review your notes, textbooks, CDs/DVDs, this review book, and any other helpful materials. A good plan is to review for a minimum of two hours each day. Studying in a group is helpful.

Testing Readiness

Answering practice questions at the end of each chapter in this text is one of the best strategies you can use to prepare for success on the WE. For the difficult questions, refer to the textbook and study that content. Pay particular attention to the Exam Alerts as well. Through review of missed practice test items, you might see a pattern of difficulty; for example, medical asepsis. If so, study that chapter in your textbook or other resource. Repeat those questions after further study to see how you progress. Keep repeating the process until you become more confident in your knowledge. Remember, answering *every* question correctly is not a realistic expectation. To successfully pass the WE, however, you must have sufficient knowledge about a variety of subjects. Use the test outline in the Introduction to help you prioritize the time you spend in reviewing the content. For example, if 35% of the examination covers nursing skills, spend more time reviewing that category than, say, legal/ethical aspects of care, which cover only 3% of the exam.

Another activity to help measure your testing readiness is to use Appendix A, "Nursing Assistant Test Cross-Reference." The appendix refers you to the questions in Practice Examinations I, II, and III that match the exam category. Review your score on the questions asked in each category to see which category requires the most study. Using the same example of medical asepsis, review your responses to questions in the Practice Examinations dealing with basic nursing skills. Pay particular attention to those questions that measure your knowledge of medical asepsis and the rationales for the correct response. Next, thoroughly review Chapter 4, "Promotion of Function and Health of Residents," and Chapter 5, "Specialized Care." Make flash cards of all terms in the chapters and use them to test your recall of the correct definitions (write the key term on one side of a note card and place the definition of the term on the back of the card). Repeat the drill until you can easily recall the terms. Continue to use Appendix A as a reference for further review of each category in the practice examinations to ensure that you do not omit any area in preparing for the exam.

Finally, repeat all practice examinations (total of 225 questions) until you score at least 80% of the questions correctly. Earning a score less than 80% means you need further study.

Use the sample 30-day review plan that follows to help organize your study time and increase your knowledge and confidence in being ready for the exam.

Four Weeks Before the Exam

Review your score on Practice Exam I. Mark those questions you missed according to the categories listed in Appendix A. Read and make notes on the chapters that help answer those missed questions. Make flash cards of all terms in those chapters, paying particular attention to the terms included in the questions you missed and those for which you have more difficulty remembering. After you read, study, and drill the flash cards, repeat the self-assessment prep questions at the end of the chapters; repeat Practice Exam I.

Three Weeks Before the Exam

Review your score on Practice Exams II and III. Mark those questions you missed according to the categories listed in Appendix A. Read and make notes on the chapters that help answer those missed questions. Make flash cards of all terms in those chapters, paying particular attention to the terms included in the questions you missed and those that you have more difficulty remembering. After you read, study, and drill the flash cards, repeat the self-assessment prep questions at the end of the chapters. Repeat Practice Exams II and III.

Two Weeks Before the Exam

Review all basic nursing skills included in Chapters 2–5, paying particular attention to direct and indirect care activities and their rationales. Review Chapter 6, "Clinical Skills Performance Checklist." Study the checkpoints for each skill until you are comfortable with them. Practice each skill with a partner, including each checkpoint and critical step, until you feel comfortable.

One Week Before the Exam

Review your notes on each chapter, all self-assessment prep questions, and both practice examinations again. Reduce your flash cards to those terms included in the missed questions, and complete another drill on those terms.

Review all instructions given to you by the testing center to ensure your understanding of where to report for the exam, what to bring (especially personal identification), and other directions.

Two Days Before the Exam

Contact the testing center if you have any questions concerning directions or other concerns. Make secure travel arrangements. If long-distance travel is necessary, plan to arrive a day early or, if not possible, at least two hours earlier than the scheduled testing time to be sure you find the testing center location without delay.

One Day Before the Exam

Study the Exam Cram page in this book, and take the page with you to the testing center site. Review the test tips and other preparation discussion in this chapter. Eat a light dinner and avoid alcohol, sleeping pills, or other drugs that might cause drowsiness or affect your thinking. Get at least eight hours of sleep. Follow the testing center's directions regarding dress or, if none available, dress comfortably in clean, tidy scrubs. Record the telephone number of the testing center in a safe, readily accessible place in the event you might need to contact the center on testing day. Prepare a snack to have on hand during testing. Make sure your personal ID and other required materials are ready. Set your clock to arrive early for the examination.

Day of the Examination

Eat a hearty but well-balanced breakfast. Drive safely to the testing center and arrive early so you can become familiar and more comfortable with the environment. Try to relax! You're prepared to pass!

Pay particular attention to Exam Alerts and the Cram Sheet in this book for last-minute, just-in-time preparation. The better prepared you are, the less stressful you will feel. Overpreparation is a good thing!

Testing Strategies

Test-taking is a skill you can learn. Based on teaching experience, those students who use test-taking techniques are more likely to succeed on their examinations. The strategies suggested here are in no way a substitute for thorough knowledge of the subject matter. If you study the review materials thoroughly and practice using the suggested strategies wisely while applying your knowledge, you can successfully pass the exam. Remember the mantra: Practice, Practice, and Practice!

Answering the Questions

The following terms help describe the key parts of a test question, commonly called *test items*:

▶ **Test item:** The question and the answer options (all possible answer choices).

▶ **Options:** All possible answers to a particular question.

▶ **Stem:** The part of the test item that asks a question or states a problem.

▶ **Multiple-choice test item:** A question offering four options. Test items are designed to measure your knowledge, attitude, or ability, not to trick you. With the multiple-choice test item, it is possible that you might not like the question or any options in the item. However, you must choose the best option available and answer the question in the best way you can.

Follow these strategies (Testing Now Tips [TNTs]) for success in answering test questions.

▶ **Take your time:** A common problem observed in test-takers is failing to read each question carefully. You might already be thinking of the right answer (option) before you finish reading the question in its entirety. Slow down and force yourself to finish reading the question before you select the option; you might be surprised that the end of the stem contains the most important information needed to select the correct option you would have otherwise missed by hurrying to record your answer. In other words, take your time!

▶ **In your own words:** Rethinking the question and answers in your own mind helps you translate the intent of the question, or what the question is asking and how you would answer it in words that mean the most to you. After you've done so, look for the option that is closest to the one you thought about; ask yourself whether that option is the best one available of the four provided. If so, go for it!

▶ **Stay under the umbrella:** Two or more options might be similar and, in your opinion, part of the answer; however, you can choose only one option. If this occurs, look for an option that contains a broader choice, an *umbrella term*, which includes those similar options and best answers to the question. For example, if the question asks you to measure the resident's physical status, you would not select option A (temperature) nor option B (pulse), nor option C (blood pressure), but option D (vital signs) that includes the other options.

▶ **Key into key terms:** Very few absolutes occur in patient care, especially when selecting the best test option. These answers are seldom, if ever correct. For that reason, look for key words in the options such as *always, never, all, only, most, none, every*, and *except*. If part of the option, choose another one!

▶ **Opposites attract:** Look for opposite options; usually, one of them is correct.

Example:

Question: When washing the perineum of the female resident, in which direction should the washcloth be applied?

  A. From the front to the back of the perineum

  B. From the middle of the perineum to the top of the perineum

  C. From any direction as long as the washcloth is wet and warm

  D. From the back of the perineum to the front

Option A is the correct answer. Option D is opposite from option A; thus, one of the two options is most likely the intended correct answer.

▶ **Feelings, feelings, feelings:** When answering a communication-type question or one requiring a response, choose the option that acknowledges or deals with the resident's feelings.

Example:

Question: A resident is upset and crying over being admitted to the nursing home. How should the nurse aide respond?

A. Tell the resident that this is normal and not to be upset.

B. Leave the resident alone to cry in private.

C. Change the subject to help the resident forget her current situation.

D. Sit with the resident and allow her to talk about her feelings.

Option D is the correct option because it acknowledges and focuses on the resident's feelings.

▶ **Safety first:** If a test item asks you for an immediate response or for deciding what to do first, choose the option that protects the resident's safety or well-being. Look for cues in the question that describe priority actions you would take; for example, "The *first* thing the nurse aide would do is"; "the *most important* step the nurse aide would take is to…"; "the *best* action the nurse aide should take is to…", "which of the following is the nurse aide's *best* response?", and so on.

▶ **Remember the face value:** Avoid reading too much into the test item. You might be tempted to remember a particular work-related or resident experience or situation that was very different from the test option you encounter. Read the item at face value, selecting the best option from the information presented.

▶ **When all else fails, choose option C:** You will encounter questions for which you have no idea of the answer. If so, and all of the preceding listed strategies fail, give it your most educated guess. No evidence exists that choosing option C is the best strategy. The point is, you will not be penalized for guessing, only for not selecting any answer at all. With a multiple-choice question, you have four chances to answer it correctly.

Taking the Clinical Skills Test

The Clinical Skills Test (CST) is the competency validation portion that most certified nurse-aide candidates dread; it is nerve racking to perform skills in front of a strange skills evaluator. A key to success on this test is, once again, to practice at least two hours each day. Review each skill you've learned so that when the performance test day arrives, you can consider it just another practice day…only for real. Practice helps build confidence; confidence decreases test anxiety.

Speaking of real, you might be required to bring along someone who can serve as the clinical actor/resident on whom you will perform selected nursing skills. Your testing actor/resident will be briefed prior to the skills examination. Each procedure will be selected by the skills evaluator. Within a specified time limit, around 30–45 minutes, you will perform at least three procedures selected from a pool of 25–30 skills. Each selected procedure will be evaluated and scored according to a skills performance checklist. Although you are not expected to perform each skill perfectly, you must **not** omit a critical step or key checkpoint of the skill, often noted with an asterisk. A critical step is defined as a step within a procedure that ensures safety of the resident (or yourself), which includes infection control. You can perform steps in a procedure out of sequence as long as infection control or another physical safety principle is not compromised. In most cases, the evaluator will not talk to you during the procedure. He/she may show you where supplies are kept and assign the skill to be performed, but, after the testing begins, the evaluator will not talk to you. The silence may be unnerving and increase your anxiety. Consider the silence "golden," in that it allows you to concentrate and perform without interruption. If you need to adjust to the silence, practice with a friend who acts as the evaluator and stress that you must have complete silence during your practice.

Another important tip regarding anxiety: BREATHE…deeply and slowly. Deep breathing will help calm your nerves and allow you to concentrate.

Self-Assessment

Before moving on to the remaining chapters of the book, complete the self-assessment Exam Prep Questions that follow to give you a baseline for focus in the upcoming chapters. See how well you recall information as you answer each question. The answer key and rationales are provided for immediate feedback. If you score 75% or better, congratulate yourself and begin reading the chapters with a smile. If you score less than 75%, congratulate yourself for completing the first step in your review journey with an honest appraisal of your knowledge, the "before" in your test readiness. Now, you can use the Exam Prep Questions as a beginning; subsequent questions at the end of each chapter and a mock written examination serve as the "after" story of your progress in preparing for the real exam. Good luck! Let's get started!

Exam Prep Questions

1. The nursing assistant can help prevent tooth decay by assisting residents to brush their teeth how often?

   ○ **A.** At least once a day

   ○ **B.** Once in the morning and once in the evening

   ○ **C.** In the morning and then after each meal

   ○ **D.** Three times at least three hours apart

2. The first step in preventing the spread of germs is which of the following?

   ○ **A.** Covering of the resident's mouth when sneezing

   ○ **B.** Handwashing

   ○ **C.** Keeping the living area clean

   ○ **D.** Emptying the trash every day

TIP

Notice the priority given in this question, that is, the *first* step. First steps often mean what you do to keep the patient safe.

---

3. All of the following are examples of the Patients' Bill of Rights except the right to which of the following?

   ○ **A.** Privacy and dignity

   ○ **B.** Confidentiality

   ○ **C.** Accept or refuse treatment

   ○ **D.** Low-cost care

4. Which of the following members of the health-care team is responsible for prescribing medical care?

   ○ **A.** Nurse

   ○ **B.** Physician or nurse practitioner

   ○ **C.** Social worker

   ○ **D.** Nurse assistant

5. When the resident requests pain medication, but the nurse appears busy, what is the appropriate action of the nursing assistant?

   ○ **A.** Report the request for pain medication to the nurse immediately.

   ○ **B.** Report the request for pain medication to the nurse when he or she appears less busy.

   ○ **C.** Tell the resident to wait for the pain medication until the pain is worse.

   ○ **D.** Tell the resident to call the nurse herself and request the pain medication.

6. The steps used to rescue a conscious choking victim that cannot cough, speak or breathe begins with

   ○ **A.** back blows

   ○ **B.** CPR

   ○ **C.** Arm elevation

   ○ **D.** Abdominal thrust

7. An observation of warmth and redness to the resident's elbow is reported as which of the following?

   ○ **A.** Jaundice

   ○ **B.** Edema

   ○ **C.** Inflammation

   ○ **D.** Cyanosis

8. The correct statement regarding religious beliefs of residents is which of the following?

   ○ **A.** Residents should not be concerned about religious beliefs.

   ○ **B.** Each resident has a right to his or her own religious beliefs.

   ○ **C.** The staff may force residents to believe as they do.

   ○ **D.** Staff or residents are not to discuss religious beliefs.

EXAM ALERT

Resident rights always take priority in the nursing home setting.

9. Which of the following residents has the greatest risk for falling?

   ○ **A.** The resident who has difficulty with balance

   ○ **B.** The hearing-impaired resident

   ○ **C.** The resident who uses a cane to ambulate

   ○ **D.** The resident who often has visitors

TIP

The previous question lists four residents at risk for falling; you must select the best choice.

10. Which of the following is appropriate for a nursing assistant working in a long-term care facility?

   ○ **A.** Preparing and administering tube feedings for a resident who is on aspiration precautions

   ○ **B.** Changing linens of an incontinent resident

   ○ **C.** Applying splints of a resident who has had a stroke

   ○ **D.** Changing the intravenous tubings of a resident receiving medication

EXAM ALERT

Remember your job duties and limitations in order to practice safely and legally according to the state's practice rules for nursing assistants.

11. An important safety step to be completed by the nursing assistant before the client is transported for a procedure is to

   ○ **A.** identify the client

   ○ **B.** ensure that the client is clean

   ○ **C.** make sure the client has eaten

   ○ **D.** position the client

12. The medical procedure used to resuscitate a client who does not have a pulse is

   ○ **A.** CPR

   ○ **B.** DPR

   ○ **C.** PPD

   ○ **D.** ADE

Answer Rationales

1. **C.** Depending on the number of meals eaten each day, teeth are to be cleaned in the morning on awakening and then after each meal. All of the other answer options do not state the proper frequency of teeth cleaning.

2. **B.** Handwashing is the most important task a nursing assistant can perform to prevent the spread of infection. Although the other answer options help prevent the spread of germs, they are not the *first* step in doing so.

3. **D.** A, B, and C are all included in the Patient's Bill of Rights.

4. **B.** The physician or nurse practitioner is the only member of the health-care team who is licensed to prescribe medical care for the residents. The nurse is responsible for carrying out both the medical plan of care prescribed by the physician as well as the nursing care plan developed by the nursing staff (answer A). The social worker in the long-term care connects the residents and family to resources available (answer C). The nursing assistant's role is a provider of direct personal care (answer D).

5. **A.** The nursing assistant is legally and ethically responsible to report pain or discomfort to the nurse as soon as possible once it is discovered. The other options represent a delay in reporting, which could lead to a change in health status or safety for the resident.

6. **A.** The steps to rescue a conscious choking victim begins with back blows and then moves to abdominal thrusts

7. **C.** Signs of inflammation are warmth, redness, and swelling. Jaundice (answer A) is a yellowing of the eyes, mucous membranes, and skin. Edema (answer B) is the collection of fluid into the subcutaneous tissue. Cyanosis (answer D) is a bluish tent to the skin from decreased oxygenation of the vessels close to the skin's surface.

8. **B.** Every resident is entitled to his or her own religious beliefs and should not feel forced to change or ignore his or her beliefs.

9. **A.** Residents who have difficulty with balance fall more often. Although the residents listed in the other options might need assistance with ambulation, they are not at the *greatest risk* for falling.

10. **B.** The changing of linens falls within the role and responsibilities of the nursing assistant; the remaining options are the role and responsibilities of the Registered and Licensed Practical Nurse.

11. **C.** The first safety step in any procedure is the proper identification of the client. It is the role of the nursing assistant to be sure they transport the right client to a procedure.

12. **A.** CPR stands for cardiopulmonary resuscitation. This procedure is used when a client is found unconscious without a pulse.

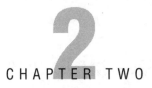

CHAPTER TWO

The Roles and Responsibilities of the Nursing Assistant

Medical Term Hotlist

ADLs	Licensed Practical Nurse (LPN)
Assault	Long-term care resident
Battery	Medical liability
Beneficence	Neglect
Caring characteristics	Negligence
Code of ethics	Non-malfeasance
Assault	Nurse Assistant/Aide
Competency	Nurse Practice Act
Confidentiality	OBRA guidelines
Continuing education	PPEs
Cultural diversity	Quality Assurance
Director of Nursing (D.O.N.)	Registered Nurse (RN)
Domestic violence	Resident's Bill of Rights
Empathy	Risk management
Ethics	Role
False imprisonment	Sexual harassment
Human Needs	Theft
Legal-ethical practice	Values

Your Role and Responsibilities

Congratulations, you have taken the first step in helping others by choosing a career in health care as a nursing assistant. Your role is to provide personal care and assistance to the elder client who might receive health-care services in a variety of settings. Although you can work in various settings, such as hospitals, clinics, physicians' offices, or clients' homes, the practice focus of this text is on the long-term care setting. If you practice in a hospital or clinical setting, you can substitute the term *patient* for all references of *resident* in this chapter. You can also substitute the title *patient care assistant* or *technician* for the title of *nursing assistant/aide*. Regardless of your practice setting or your title, your job or position description outlines your responsibilities and duties in detail. The most important tasks you perform are direct personal care of the client referred to as the resident.

Job Responsibilities

Tasks listed on your job description can vary from one facility to another but often include personal care, including, but not limited to

▶ **Activities of daily living (ADLs):** Personal care activities performed by residents every day, which include bathing, grooming, dressing, eating and hydrating, toileting, ambulating, and exercising.

▶ **Measurement and client observation:** Measuring, recording, and reporting resident vital signs (temperature, pulse, respiration, and blood pressure), height and weight, intake and output, meal consumption, changes in resident's condition, collecting laboratory specimens, and applying resident restraints.

▶ **Procedures outlined in facility procedure manual and performed under the supervision of a licensed nurse:** Performing skills including instilling enemas; applying non-sterile dressings; applying ice packs; attending to skin and oral needs; and admitting, transferring, and discharging patients.

▶ **Infection control:** Adhering to facility care standards; that is, preventing and isolating client infection through handwashing, care and handling of contaminated objects, isolation procedures, and observing and reporting environmental situations that might spread infection.

▶ **Assisting with client ambulation, movement, and exercise:** Lifting, moving, and transporting residents from one position to another, from one room to another, or from one facility to another. Assisting the resident to maintain or regain normal range of motion and body strength, and assisting physical exercise to maintain musculoskeletal function and general well-being.

▶ **Environmental care and safety:** Making residents' living conditions as comfortable and safe as possible by keeping the residents' rooms clean and tidy, making beds and arranging residents' furniture, adjusting room temperature and lighting, removing potential safety hazards or sources of personal injury, such as spills or objects left on the floor, removing refuse and caring for plants, and performing CPR and resident evacuation in case of fire or other environmental threats.

▶ **Communication:** Verbal or written communication with clients, visitors, and health-care team members; observing and recording resident care or information; and answering the telephone and taking messages.

Other Tasks and Duties

Other tasks and duties that fall under the responsibility of the nursing assistant include the following:

▶ Protecting residents' rights, privacy, confidentiality, and dignity

▶ Following safety rules, adhering to legal and ethical standards of care

▶ Complying with all agency policies

▶ Promoting client safety and well-being

▶ Participating in facility efforts to provide quality care and performance improvement activities

▶ Continuing staff education

▶ Performing post-mortem procedures

Job Limitations

You must work under the direction of a licensed nurse or doctor. Your job responsibilities are limited to those specified in your job description. Limitations often include giving medications (includes applying prescription skin creams, lotions, or ointments), taking orders from a doctor, and performing any procedures prohibited by law or by the employing facility. When in doubt about performing any function or task for which you are unfamiliar or unsure, consult your immediate supervisor. In medicine, the adage "Do no harm" applies to your practice as well.

Personal Qualities

Honesty is one of the most important qualities you can bring to your job. Second only to knowing your job well and being accountable for what you do is being truthful in your interactions with others. Accepting your own limitations is another example of being truthful. These qualities are essential to effective, lawful practice.

Caring means having a sincere regard for the safety and well-being of all residents in your care and being willing to care for them and about them. You can be the most skillful nursing assistant in the facility, but if you do not care about what happens to the residents, you are in the wrong job. The time you spend with residents other than the time required is a good way to evaluate your caring characteristics. Spending time with residents is only one way to evaluate caring behaviors, but it is an effective job performance measure. The following caring characteristics are the hallmark of the exemplary employee:

▶ *Being considerate* of others, both residents and coworkers, is very important if you are to be an effective nursing assistant.

▶ *Being empathetic*; that is, seeing yourself in others' situations without pitying them is also a very important attribute you must possess. Consideration for other peoples' feelings is also an important personal quality for effective practice. This means being aware of the effect of what you say and how you say it; cooperating with coworkers to help support them and the facility when short-staffed is another example of being considerate.

▶ *Having respect for other people* is important, especially when their values, culture, language, or beliefs differ from your own. Honesty, empathy, sincerity, and caring behaviors are all part of legal and ethical practice—basic but crucial expectations of your employer. Values, culture, and language considerations are included in subsequent chapters.

▶ *Dependability* is a basic expectation of your employer. Coming to work when scheduled and on time demonstrates your commitment to your job and to the residents. Doing what you commit to do and doing it consistently also help to demonstrate your dependability.

▶ *Flexibility* and dependability go hand in hand. Despite the best assignment plan, "stuff happens," meaning you might be reassigned to another unit or group of residents or staff you do not know. You must be able to accept this normal disruption in your work schedule and make the best of the situation.

▶ *Accountability* is a key quality you bring to your work. You must care for all residents in a variety of conditions and situations that you have been prepared to handle, and you are expected to perform your duties in the way you have been trained to perform them. Should you have any questions or concerns about your assignment, you should discuss them privately with your supervisor.

▶ *Self-responsibility* is required for your own health and safety. Wearing personal protective equipment (PPE), using effective body mechanics when moving and lifting clients, maintaining a safe workspace, organizing your work to conserve energy, and maintaining a healthy life style are examples of those actions you must take to protect yourself and promote your own well-being.

The Nursing Assistant as a Member of the Health-Care Team

You are one of the most important members of the health-care team, working with other nursing staff as well as technicians, therapists, health-care providers (physicians or nurse practitioners), dieticians, social workers, the clergy, support staff, and administration to help meet the mission of the facility whose goal is to provide the very best care possible to all residents. Each of the following nursing staff members contributes to the well-being of the residents:

▶ **Registered Nurse (RN):** The RN is responsible for carrying out both the medical plan of care prescribed by the physician as well as the nursing care plan developed by the nursing staff. The RN assesses each resident and modifies the nursing care as needed to help meet the patient's needs. The RN also works with other therapists and staff to ensure the well-being of each resident. He or she assigns unlicensed assistive staff members to each day's personal care activities and supervises the work. The RN works under the supervision of the Director of Nursing and is accountable for his or her practice according to the state's nurse practice act, which outlines the practice competencies as well as limitations of the practice. The RN might supervise other RNs, LPNs, or unlicensed assistive personnel (UAPs).

▶ **Licensed Practical Nurse (LPN):** Like the RN, the LPN carries out the medical and nursing plans of care for assigned residents but works under the supervision of the RN. The LPN performs treatments, administers medications, and documents care given according to a prescribed scope of practice set by the board of nursing or other licensing agency of the state in which the LPN practices. The LPN might supervise UAPs as well. His or her duties can be expanded with additional training and credentialing.

▶ **Nursing Assistant/Nurse Aide (CNA) or Patient Care Assistant/Technician (PCA/PCT):** The CNA (or PCA/PCT) performs care and carries out duties under the supervision of the RN or LPN. The CNA (or PCA/PCT) is in a unique position as a *first responder* at the bedside. He or she becomes the eyes, ears, and hands of the licensed nurse, often being the first team member to identify resident needs and problems that can become life threatening.

As a CNA, you spend more time with residents than any other team member. Because of your close interactions with residents, you befriend them and become their advocates, meaning you communicate their needs when they might not be able to.

You can also serve as the first line of defense for residents in situations that might threaten their health or well-being. For example, you will often be the first team member to notice a change in the resident's vital signs that can signal an infection. You might also be the first to notice a skin irritation, a warning sign of a developing bedsore. Because you spend so much time with a resident, you might be the first team member to notice subtle changes in behavior that could point to a serious infection. These are only a few examples of the unique role you play on the health-care team.

Other Team Members

▶ **Dietician (RD):** Licensed professional who plans client's diet according to physician order to assure the client receives required nutrients to maintain or restore health.

▶ **Physical Therapist (RPT):** Licensed professional who follows physician order to maintain musculoskeletal function to help ensure client mobility and other physical abilities to promote physical well-being.

▶ **Respiratory Therapist (RT):** Licensed professional who carries out physician order to maintain, promote, or regain respiratory functions. Therapy may include medications via aerosol delivery system.

▶ **Social Worker (LMHP or LSW):** Licensed professional who provides guidance to secure social services (housing, insurance, agency assistance) to promote psychosocial health; secures necessary social assistance to promote, maintain, or gain social independence for clients.

Being a Team Player

As a team member, you carry out duties assigned to you by the RN or LPN. While you are responsible for completing assignments for specific residents in a timely manner, you also assist other team members with their assignments when you have completed your own or when urgent help is needed. Cooperating willingly to assist coworkers is an expectation of any employer but is particularly important in the long-term care facility. An isolated approach to your work is not only unmanageable but also potentially harmful to you and the residents. An example of working alone is lifting, moving, or assisting the resident to ambulate by yourself. The resident will feel safer if two or more staff members assist with this task. You also protect yourself, other workers, and the resident from injury by asking for help when you need it.

Working well with others is a hallmark of an efficient and effective nursing assistant. Your coworkers will more likely offer to help you if you assist them with enthusiasm and a can-do approach. Your supervisor will welcome your cooperation with assignments when carried out cheerfully and to the best of your ability. If you have a concern about an assignment or with a situation involving your coworker's approach to cooperation and teamwork, discuss it privately with your immediate supervisor.

Being a team player also means being able to accept constructive criticism, especially from your supervisor. Listening to your superior's feedback without being defensive helps you to improve your performance and contribute to your job satisfaction. Always follow the facility's chain of command when resolving work-related issues, especially for work conflicts or other disagreements that are bound to occur. It is important for you to consult with your supervisor about any situations that will potentially interfere with resident welfare or that will compromise your own values and well-being.

Communication and Interpersonal Skills Needed for Effective CNA Practice

Being able to express yourself verbally and in writing is a skill you learn and apply throughout your health-care career. Likewise, forming positive working relationships with your coworkers and building effective interpersonal relationships with residents are essential elements in effective CNA practice. Communication skills involve listening, responding, and documenting what residents tell you about themselves and their unique needs. Active listening—that is, listening to residents without being distracted by your own thoughts—is key to acknowledging them as worthy human beings who deserve your attention. This skill is called listening with a "third" ear. Your skill in observing what is omitted in conversation with residents will cue you to their unexpressed needs.

Verbal communication skills include speaking clearly at a level residents can understand—that is, avoiding medical jargon; asking open-ended questions that discourage a yes/no response; using phrases to encourage further exploration of thoughts and feelings: "Oh?," "Tell me more," and so on; and clarifying the message you receive: "Let me see if I understand what you mean…," "Is this what I hear you say…?," and so on.

Communication barriers can occur in practice. Try to avoid the following pitfalls when communicating with the resident: asking close-ended questions that prompt a yes/no answer; speaking "over the resident's head," using medical terms or other language that he or she cannot understand; and responding to him or her with advice, criticism, or sarcasm. Responses to the resident that begins with "You should/shouldn't…" or "Why?" are not only demeaning but encourage defensiveness and limit further communication. This reluctance to communicate can be hazardous for the resident and a detriment to an effective relationship with you.

It is important to recognize communication barriers that interfere with effective interpersonal relationships with residents and to seek guidance and help from your supervisor to solve any communication problem you might encounter. Use an interpreter or family member to assist you in talking with the resident whose primary language is not English, and be patient with the resident who struggles to understand your language. Cultural barriers can also interfere with effective communication, especially if the resident's culture is very different from your own. Nonverbal gestures like avoiding eye contact might be viewed by the resident as offensive or disrespectful. Other cues to barriers include personal space (for example, standing too close to the resident), smiling or other facial expressions that do not match the verbal message, and your conversational tone or body posture. For example, smiling when talking to a resident might imply your agreement. At the same time, standing with your arms crossed over your chest and leaning away from the resident is a message that you, indeed, do not agree with him or her. At best, this message is confusing if not disrespectful. Admitting your own limitations and working to improve your communication skills are positive steps to building meaningful relationships.

Equally important to effective interpersonal relationships with residents is the need to maintain resident safety through clear communication. Countless stories abound regarding accidental resident injury or neglect that resulted from failure to communicate. Examples include failure to explain the dangers of walking without assistance for residents with mobility problems, misunderstanding or lack of sufficient information for family members regarding restrictions to their resident's diabetic diet that led to hyperglycemia, or residents becoming upset with a change in their care plan due to faulty interpretation of the nursing staff's instructions. Barriers to communication also include those linked to the senses (vision, hearing, and other sensory deficits). Speaking clearly, slowly, and directly to the hearing-impaired resident is important to ensure his or her understanding of your verbal communication. Offering large-print reading materials or other assistance to the resident who is visually impaired is equally important. Some residents have a decreased sensation to pain and temperature changes. Specific details regarding working with impaired residents are covered in subsequent chapters.

Reporting conversations between you and the resident is also important to maintain his or her safety and well-being. This includes changes in resident condition, his or her specific requests, concerns or evaluations regarding care, safety considerations, and other pertinent observations.

Recording observations, measurements, and personal care of the resident is an important nursing assistant function. Charting and other resident documentation requires knowledge of medical terminology and abbreviations, proper spelling and grammar, and basic computation skills. For example, measuring intake and output requires mathematics/addition with results expressed in milliliters, not household measures. Recording "I & O" is acceptable terminology for charting. Factual recording is required because your personal opinion has no purpose in communication. Although observation is the first step to assuring resident safety, you must record and report any resident responses to care or change in condition promptly to your supervisor. Consult your supervisor for help with documentation to ensure completeness, objectivity, and accuracy. Remember, you can never overcommunicate!

Legal and Ethical Considerations in Practice

Your job description is based on laws and rules for nursing assistant practice set by government agencies. As long as you follow those rules when carrying out your duties and observe the law, you are not liable for your performance. Liability means being responsible for providing care according to an accepted standard. If you perform duties outside your job description or perform appropriate duties incorrectly that result in harm to a resident, you can be found liable. Examples of liable acts include the following:

- **Abuse:** A threat or actual physical or mental harm to a resident.

- **Aiding and abetting:** Participating in an unlawful act or observing it and not reporting it. For example, observing sexual harassment of a resident and not reporting it.

- **Assault:** Threat or actual touching of a resident without permission.

- **Battery:** Unlawful personal violence toward a resident; for example, bathing a resident without his or her permission.

- **False imprisonment:** Preventing a resident from moving freely about, with or without force, against the resident's wishes.

- **Invasion of privacy:** Failing to keep the resident's affairs confidential or exposing the resident's body when performing care.

- **Involuntary seclusion:** Keeping a resident isolated from others as a form of punishment.

- **Neglect:** Accidently or deliberately ignoring the needs of a resident that results in harm or injury.

- **Negligence:** Either neglecting to act in the manner in which you were taught, or omitting care or performing care incorrectly that results in harm to a resident.

- **Theft:** Taking something that does not belong to you.

Resident Rights

In 1973 the American Hospital Association (AHA) issued a policy for all patients called "A Patient's Bill of Rights." Soon after that publication, a guide for long-term residents was developed, called "Resident's Bill of Rights." Although both bills are similar, the Resident's Bill of Rights contains additional considerations for residents in long-term care settings. By law, all nursing homes must have written policies describing residents' rights and must make them available to any resident. The following outlines the issues addressed in the bill of rights; namely, that every resident has the right to the following:

- **Be informed about the facility's services and charges:** The services of the nursing home and all charges involved with the services should be made available and fully explained to every resident. Likewise, charges that are not covered by Medicare or Medicaid should also be included in the notice of services; this includes those services not covered by the basic charges for facility rates.

▶ **Be informed about one's medical condition:** Unless the physician notes in the medical record that to be informed of his or her medical condition is not in his or her best interest, every resident deserves to be apprised of his or her medical condition. Be truthful with your answers to residents' questions about their condition, being careful to inform them of what you observe only. An example of this is answering the resident's questions about vital signs or output. The RN or doctor should answer the resident's medical condition questions because you cannot answer medical questions that you have not been prepared to answer. It is your responsibility to report the resident's request for information to your supervisor.

▶ **Participate in the plan of care:** Every resident must have the opportunity to partici-pate in his or her plan of care or to refuse care or treatment. Despite your belief that a procedure or care activity will be helpful to residents, be very careful that you do not force them to participate against their wishes. This includes assisting other staff to do the same. Failure to observe this resident right is an example of assault, battery, and invasion of privacy.

▶ **Choose one's own physician:** Every resident has the right to determine his or her own physician and pharmacy. Remember, your personal opinion is unimportant in this situation. Refer the resident to the RN or social worker for assistance.

▶ **Manage one's own personal finances:** Residents can manage their own finances or appoint someone else (power of attorney) to manage them. If authorized by the resident to manage funds, the manager must report the resident's financial status as directed and provide all receipts for business transactions. Avoid handling the resident's money or valuables (for example, inventory of personal items when admitted to the facility) without a witness.

▶ **Privacy, dignity, and respect:** Privacy, dignity, and respect for each resident are of the utmost importance. Privacy includes visitation for married couples. Close the door to assure couples are alone and are not interrupted; knock before entering the room. Each caregiver must knock before entering the patient's/resident's room EVERY TIME the caregiver enters. Remember, the room is the patient's/client's personal space and, thus, must be respected. Part of providing respect is to address the resident by his or her formal name until given permission to use a first name.

▶ **Use one's own clothing and possessions:** Unless hazardous, or potentially infringing on other residents' rights, each resident has the right to wear his or her own clothing and use his or her own possessions.

▶ **Be free from abuse and restraints:** Residents must be protected from mental and physical abuse, which can include unauthorized use of restraints. Except as authorized in writing by a physician for a specified and limited time, or when necessary to protect the individual from hurting himself/herself or others, residents must be free from chemical or physical restraints that cause them to be unable to freely move about.

Mental abuse refers to any threat to the resident's psychological well-being that results in psychological or emotional distress. This can include financial exploitation or verbal assault. Depriving residents of any of their rights listed here is considered mental abuse.

Physical abuse includes hitting or rough handling of a resident. Withholding food or fluids or failure to change a wet bed are forms of physical abuse. Sexual abuse is a form of physical abuse and involves threats or physical contact for sexual favor or control. Fondling or inappropriately touching a resident, rape, sexual assault, or sexual molestation are examples of sexual abuse. Sexual harassment, or making unwelcomed sexually explicit or implied statements to residents, is abusive and could become grounds for resident grievance or legal action.

Watch for signs or other clues of resident abuse that might include the following:

▶ Skin tears or bruises, especially in the genital area

▶ Frequent crying or periods of sadness or withdrawal

▶ Personality changes

▶ Refusal to carry out ADLs

▶ Fear of touch

▶ Anxiety or nervousness

▶ Refusal of certain visitors, including spouse or family members

You have a moral, ethical, and legal duty to report suspicion of abuse. Be as factual as possible, avoiding assumptions and expressing personal opinions about what you observe. Do not worry if your suspicions are unfounded. Your sincere attempt to protect the resident outweighs any fears you might have. In all cases, follow the facility policy for reporting abuse concerns. Abuse hotlines might also be available for reporting suspicions of abuse. An Ombudsmen Committee might also be available as a source for investigating abuse complaints. An Ombudsmen Committee is a group of concerned citizens, usually appointed by the state governor, to investigate all complaints of abuse. The committee members are not affiliated with a health-care facility. The originator of the abuse complaint, whether a fellow citizen or a health-care provider, is kept confidential.

▶ **Grievance without retaliation:** Residents should be able to express concerns, make recommendations about facility services or care, and consult with outside sources to resolve conflicts involved in their care without fear of criticism, discrimination, or other acts of vengeance by the facility or its staff.

▶ **Be discharged or transferred only for specific reasons:** Residents might be transferred or discharged from a facility only for medical reasons, for their welfare or the welfare of other residents, or for nonpayment, which excludes becoming Medicaid eligible. If transfer or discharge is planned, the resident or representative must be notified in writing within 30 days of the change.

▶ **Access to**

- ▶ Receive or refuse any visitor (includes family members)

- ▶ Visiting hours, posted in public places

- ▶ Confidential communication with visitors, including help with personal, social, or legal services

- ▶ Claim own rights and benefits through consultation with others for the purpose of legal action, organizational activity, or other forms of representation

Ethics

Ethics is often linked with legalities when determining right and lawful behavior in health care. Ethics is a branch of philosophy dealing with the good, bad, right, and wrong thing to do in human interactions and the principles that help guide professionals in terms of what ought to be done in certain situations. Ethical principles, or standards, help guide you in your work. Examples cited include *beneficence*, or doing good for others. Confidentiality is another principle that you follow to keep residents' matters private. *Nonmaleficence*, or "do no harm," underscores the need to not cause undo harm to a resident, or to provide safe and effective care. Veracity, or truthfulness, means speaking the truth consistently and dependably.

Health-care professionals such as nurses adhere to a published code of ethics, which admonishes them to practice in an ethical manner at all times. Such guiding principles help form a practice framework on which nurses can build. A description of ethical behavior is to "do the right thing when nobody else is looking." This could be evidenced by refusing to accept money, gifts, or favors from residents or their families; avoiding shortcuts in job performance; maintaining a positive attitude about the facility; and treating residents' belongings with care.

Ethical problems occur when your "inner ethical voice" conflicts with a situation that causes you to struggle with the right course of action to maintain your values, often reflected in ethical principles. Ethical dilemmas abound in today's world, especially in health care. Specific examples of ethical dilemmas regarding residents in long-term care mirror those of clients in other health-care settings, such as quality-of-life issues, death and dying, access to health care, and euthanasia. Solutions can become quite weighty but need not be solved alone. As a health team member, you can seek guidance from your supervisor and other professionals, including the clergy, to sort out all available alternatives in an ethical situation. Use your resources wisely in this regard and remember that you are not experiencing the situation alone.

Exam Prep Questions

Directions: Select the best response to each question.

1. A nursing assistant who is threatening to apply a restraint to a resident is an example of which of the following?

   ○ **A.** Assault

   ○ **B.** False imprisonment

   ○ **C.** Invasion of privacy

   ○ **D.** Battery

2. Which of the following is an example of verbal communication?

   ○ **A.** Touch

   ○ **B.** Facial expressions

   ○ **C.** Body language

   ○ **D.** Speech

3. Which of the following statements describes the role of the nursing assistant?

   ○ **A.** Performs the list of activities an employer expects the nursing assistant to carry out once hired

   ○ **B.** Provides personal care and assistance as needed

   ○ **C.** Performs work for moral or ethical reasons

   ○ **D.** Conducts actions out of a sense for what is right or wrong

4. The nursing assistant obtained a resident's temperature as 102°F. Which of the following is the nursing assistant's next action?

   ○ **A.** Continue with obtaining the vital signs of the other residents and report the temperature to the first nurse the nursing assistant encounters.

   ○ **B.** Ask another nursing assistant to report the temperature to the nurse assigned to the resident.

   ○ **C.** Come back to the resident and repeat the temperature after collecting all the vital signs of the other residents.

   ○ **D.** Report the temperature to the nurse assigned to the resident immediately.

5. Which of the following demonstrates dignity and respect for the resident?

   ○ **A.** The nursing assistant addresses the resident by his or her first name.

   ○ **B.** After hugging the resident, the nursing assistant calls the resident "honey" or "dear."

    ○ **C.** The nursing assistant uses the resident's proper name and title whenever addressing the resident.

    ○ **D.** The staff calls the resident by a nickname given by the staff.

6. Which team member is responsible for planning the meals for the residents?

    ○ **A.** Orderly

    ○ **B.** Nursing assistant

    ○ **C.** Nurse

    ○ **D.** Dietician

7. The nursing assistant assigned to obtain vital signs for a group of residents omits taking the vital signs of one of the residents. When the nurse inquires as to the resident's missing vital signs, the nurse assistant admits forgetting the resident. This is an example of which of the following?

    ○ **A.** Accountability

    ○ **B.** Flexibility

    ○ **C.** Dependability

    ○ **D.** Respectability

8. A resident's neighbor inquires about the condition of the resident. Which of the following actions is a demonstration of confidentiality by the nursing assistant?

    ○ **A.** Share with the neighbor the condition of the resident.

    ○ **B.** Inform the neighbor that you cannot share that information.

    ○ **C.** Suggest that the neighbor go to the nurse's station with you and view the chart.

    ○ **D.** Ask the neighbor to step out into the hall to share the condition of the resident.

9. Which of the following ways can a nursing assistant demonstrate empathy?

    ○ **A.** Putting others ahead of self

    ○ **B.** Sharing of emotions with residents

    ○ **C.** Imagining self in the place of others

    ○ **D.** Going the extra mile for someone

10. When a nursing assistant enter a client's room without knocking first, the assistant is demonstrating a lack of privacy for the client.

    ○ **A.** True

    ○ **B.** False

11. A nursing assistant upholds client confidentiality by

     ○ **A.** sharing information that is needed for the purpose of the client's care.

     ○ **B.** verifying with visitors everything the client tells you.

     ○ **C.** asking the client personal information that is interesting to know.

     ○ **D.** sharing with other nursing assistants when a client reveals a funny story about his or her life.

12. When a nursing assistant witnesses a health-care team member sexually harassing a resident but does not report it is considered

     ○ **A.** An invasion of privacy

     ○ **B.** Negligence

     ○ **C.** Aiding and abetting

     ○ **D.** Battery

Answer Rationales

1. **A.** Assault is the threat or actual touching of a resident without permission. False imprisonment is to prevent a resident from moving freely about, with or without force (answer B). Invasion of privacy would be failing to keep a resident's affairs confidential or exposing the resident's body when performing care (answer C). Battery is the unlawful personal violence toward a resident (answer D).

2. **D.** Speech and sign language are forms of verbal communication. The other selections are all forms of nonverbal communication. Nonverbal communication includes the process of sending and receiving messages without the use of words.

3. **B.** Providing personal care and assistance as needed describes the role of the nursing assistant. Performing the list of activities an employer expects the nursing assistant to carry out once hired (answer A) is the definition of the responsibilities of the nursing assistant. Performing work for moral or ethical reasons (answer C) is an example of ethical reasoning. Conducting actions out of a sense for what is right or wrong (answer D) is the definition for obligation.

4. **D.** The nursing assistant is legally and ethically responsible to report abnormal data to the nurse as soon as possible. The options in A, B, and C represent a delay in reporting, which might lead to a change in health status or safety for the resident.

5. **C.** To maintain a resident's dignity and respect for him or her as a person, only formal names and titles should be used at all times and in all situations. The options in A, B, and D are ways of addressing close friends and family.

6. **D.** The dietician is responsible for planning the meals for the residents. The orderly (answer A) and nurse assistant (answer B) are responsible for the provision of care and assistance to residents. The nurse's part as a member of the health-care team is to carry out the physician's prescription and nursing goals (answer C).

7. **A.** This is an example of accountability, even when admitting that you did not properly carry out your duties. Flexibility (answer B) is your ability to adapt to the situation. Dependability (answer C) is a basic expectation set by your employer, and the nursing assistant demonstrates this by his or her commitment to the job and to the residents. Responsibility (answer D) is the ability to fulfill duties and expectations in your role as a nursing assistant.

8. **B.** Confidentiality is keeping the resident's medical information private. The options in A, C, and D violate the resident's right to confidentiality.

9. **C.** Empathy is putting self in the place of someone else to try to understand what he or she might be experiencing without pitying him or her. Putting others ahead of self (answer A) demonstrates caring. Sharing of emotions with residents (answer B) demonstrates sharing by friends and is not appropriate for a professional relationship. Going the extra mile for someone (answer D) is an example of respect.

10. **True.** The nursing assistant is to provide privacy and respect for the client by knocking on the door and waiting to be given permission to enter before going in the room each time the assistant needs to enter the room.

11. **A.** Confidentiality is the act of keeping private matters of the client private, not sharing information with anyone who does not need to know it for the care of the client. In answers B, C, and D, the nursing assistant is sharing a client's private information with persons who do not need the information to care for the client.

12. **C.** Participating in an unlawful act or observing it and not reporting it is the definition of aiding and abetting an unlawful act.

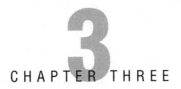

CHAPTER THREE

Promotion of Health and Safety

Medical Term Hotlist

Adverse Drug Events (ADEs)

AIDS

Airborne transmission

Antisepsis

Bacteria

Biohazardous waste

Blood-borne pathogens

Communicable disease

Contact isolation

Contagion

Droplet transmission

Hepatitis B virus (HBV)

Hepatitis C virus (HCV)

Infection control

Isolation

Medical asepsis

Microorganisms

MRSA (methicillin-resistant Staphylococcus aureus)

OSHA guidelines

Pathogen

Personal Protective Equipment (PPE)

Risk management

Scabies

Shingles

Standard precautions

Sterile

Tuberculosis (TB)

Virus

VRE (vancomycin-resistant Enterococcus)

Review of Body Systems Affected by Aging

Health means that all systems of the body are working normally. *Wellness* is defined by each person who takes into account how he or she views his or her health and happiness, often described as the sense of well-being, or outlook on the future.

The human body is made up of systems—a group of organs, each with a specific makeup and function. Each organ within a system works with other organs to keep the body healthy. For example, the stomach and intestines are organs of the gastrointestinal system whose function is to take in, digest, and eliminate food and fluids to keep the body nourished. Body systems are the backdrop for this chapter as you review *disease*, the absence of wellness. More important is your role and responsibility to promote resident health and safety while helping to prevent the spread of disease.

As residents age, their body systems do not function as fully as when they were younger. This "wear-and-tear" theory of stress on each body system makes residents more susceptible to disease or injury. *Immunity*, the ability to ward off disease, might also decrease due to the natural aging process. Certain diseases can also affect immunity and medical treatment, such as cancer and the drugs used to treat it.

Although health and well-being vary among residents, all share the following common, age-related changes for which they must adapt:

- ▶ Risk for chronic illness
- ▶ Changes in mobility
- ▶ Decreased vision and hearing
- ▶ Decreased ability to sense pain
- ▶ Change in sleep habits

It is a myth that healthy older adults, often called elders, lose intellectual abilities; that is, their wisdom, judgment, and common sense. However, research proves that elders over age 60 might have a slight loss of short-term memory, mathematical calculations, word construction, and abstract thinking. Although a bit slower, elders can learn new skills.

Normal aging does not necessarily affect mobility. Age-related changes, however, could affect muscle strength, flexibility, and stability. Joint changes caused by chronic conditions, such as arthritis or muscle tremors from Parkinson's disease, can also affect the ability to stand, stoop, and walk. When mobility is affected by aging, elders risk falling, which can lead to injury requiring hospitalization. Many elders might never regain fully functional mobility. Injuries from falls are the second leading cause of death in elders over age 65 and are the leading cause of death for those 85 years and older.

The ability to see clearly and at long distances declines with age. Elders have difficulty seeing well in dimly lit areas or at night, which puts them at high risk for falls as well. Cataracts, or a clouding of the lens of the eye, can also contribute to the risk for falls. Unless treated early, glaucoma, a chronic disease affecting the optic nerve of the eye, can put elders at risk for blindness.

Hearing loss is a normal part of aging, especially if persons are exposed to high noise levels at a young age. Meniere's, a chronic disease affecting the inner ear, can put elders at risk for falls due to dizziness, which interferes with normal movement and ambulation.

Older adults might ignore signs and symptoms of illness or injury due to a less than normal ability to feel pain. This can occur in elders with diabetes, who might develop an open sore or a cut on their foot or lower leg but not feel any discomfort until the injured area becomes infected.

Risk factors for chronic illness (those factors affecting particular persons and not others) can also contribute to illness. These include cultural, racial, and ethnic factors. For example, diabetes is higher among African Americans, Hispanics, Native Americans, and Native Alaskans than for white Americans. Likewise, obesity is becoming a public health crisis for North American populations compared to persons living in other countries. Access to health care, or lack of it, affects how timely persons in one cultural or ethnic group seek treatment for an illness, which, if left untreated, becomes a chronic health problem. Hypertension, or high blood pressure, is an example of a condition that, if left untreated, can lead to a stroke. Economic status also can be considered a risk factor if an individual does not have health insurance and cannot afford health care.

Cultural or religious beliefs might prevent individuals from participating in certain traditional health-care practices. Instead of seeking care from a physician, for example, they rely on others in the community who can provide care through alternative medical therapies or folk remedies.

Other chronic diseases, such as dementia, Alzheimer's disease, circulation problems, or mental confusion caused by arteriosclerosis or the effects of a stroke, can all affect thinking and reasoning processes. These chronic conditions can put elders at risk for injury.

Communicable Diseases and Their Effect on Health

Diseases can sicken an individual alone or can be *communicable, or contagious*, in nature, meaning they can spread from one person to another. In the case of long-term residents, communicable diseases or infections are transmitted by a *pathogen* (disease-causing microorganism) that can infect many residents who live in the same location. Pathogens can include bacteria, viruses, fungi, and parasites. A common bacterial pathogen that is particularly worrisome in the long-term care setting is *methicillin-resistant Staphylococcus aureus*, often referred to as *MRSA*. MRSA is an infection of the skin that can spread to the blood stream and become life threatening. MSRA is resistant to certain antibiotics (drugs that kill bacteria), such as Methicillin. It is difficult to kill and, if left untreated or a chronic infection develops, MRSA can strike an entire population of residents. MRSA is also becoming a major health problem in the general community.

Other infectious diseases can infect long-term residents, such as tuberculosis (TB), a bacterial illness; influenza, a viral infection; pneumonia, of viral or bacterial origin; or the most commonly spread virus, the common cold. Pathogens causing these illnesses can enter the body by *contamination* through direct contact (for example, blood or body fluids or open wounds) or by droplet (for example, inhaled through the air). Specific organ systems become infected, which give rise to signs and symptoms indicating an acute infection or illness. Unfortunately, residents often become contagious before their symptoms appear. Signs and symptoms of infection include but are not limited to fever, chills, elevated white blood cell count, wounds containing a strong odor or drainage, local heat, and redness around a skin sore or other body lesion, a general sense of not feeling well (*malaise*), and mental confusion.

Infections or conditions involving the skin can become contagious through direct contact. Examples of these conditions are *scabies*, a skin infestation by a tiny mite that causes a rash and intense itching, and *shingles*, a skin condition caused by a virus that attacks a nerve path, which causes pain and disability. The drainage from open shingles blisters can infect others by direct contact.

The following is a quick review of common terms regarding communicable disease:

- **Antisepsis:** The prevention of sepsis by preventing or slowing the growth of disease-causing germs.

- **Infection control:** Measures to prevent or limit infection; control methods vary depending on the type of germ and how it is spread.

- **Isolation:** An attempt to limit the spread of disease by its mode of transmission (for example, respiratory precautions for a tuberculosis patient).

- **Medical asepsis:** Procedures to reduce the number of germs in the environment.

- **Pathogen:** Disease-causing microorganism or germ.

- **Sepsis:** Putrefaction; infection. System-wide response to a specific infection.

Role of the Nursing Assistant to Prevent the Spread of Communicable Diseases

You play an important role in reinforcing the nurse's teaching plan regarding infection control for residents. You can help explain to residents the reasons for limiting their exposure to other residents who are ill, why they must not share equipment or supplies with other residents, how they can avoid cross-contamination when visiting other residents, how to practice good handwashing and self-care practices, and so on. Residents' families must also be included in the teaching plan to help ensure residents' health.

You must take responsibility for your own health as well as that of the residents. Following the facility's policies and procedures for health screening, including TB surveillance, immunizations and health history, not working while you are ill, practicing effective hand hygiene, and other infection control measures are essential for safe practice.

The following sections outline the infection control guidelines, procedures, and precautions you must follow to guard residents and yourself from infection.

Medical Asepsis

Adhere to specific facility policies and procedures regarding infection control when providing care for residents, which applies to patients in acute care facilities as well.

- **Use of standard precautions:** The following standards set guidelines to prevent and control disease as recommended by the Center for Disease Control (CDC):

  - **Hand hygiene and contamination:**

    Wash hands when visibly dirty or contaminated with blood or other body fluids.

    Wash hands with plain soap and hot water using friction for at least 30 seconds.

    Wash hands before eating and after using the restroom, before and after entering a resident's room, and before and after touching a resident's belongings or personal equipment.

    Remember, reinforce handwashing with each resident, encouraging them to wash their hands as needed to prevent the spread of germs.

TIP

Handwashing is the most effective precaution used to control infections in residents and staff. It is now recommended that health-care workers sing the Happy Birthday song twice while washing hands before and after every resident contact.

Apply hand lotion to limit breaks in the skin from frequent handwashing and antiseptic product applications.

CAUTION

Follow agency policy for approved lotions. To help avoid contamination of the lotion, do not use lotions from large containers.

Keep nails natural (no artificial nails), with tips trimmed to less than 1/4 inch; no nail polish or decals allowed.

Apply an antiseptic hand-rub product.

> **NOTE**
>
> For optimum effect when using hand sanitizers, apply generous amounts to hands, applying friction with laced fingers, and let the sanitizer dry completely before touching the resident.

▶ **Hand hygiene in all other clinical situations:** All clinical situations include direct contact with the resident and the resident's personal articles.

Gloves:

Wear gloves when in contact with blood or other potentially infectious materials, mucous membranes, and non-intact skin.

Change gloves during resident care as needed when moving from a contaminated body site to a clean body site.

Remove gloves when resident care is completed.

> **CAUTION**
>
> Change gloves with each new resident contact.

Wash hands after removing gloves.

Mask, Eye Protection, Face Shield, Gowns

The risk of being splashed with blood and body fluids (including tears, saliva, semen, vaginal secretions, urine, or fluid drawn from body cavities) is higher in the acute care setting, but splashes can occur in any setting and should be avoided. Wear a mask, eye protection, or gown if you risk exposure. To protect against airborne contamination, wear a mask as directed by the specific *isolation* procedure required in your facility. You should also protect yourself when such a disease is suspected but not diagnosed. Chapter 6, "Clinical Skills Performance Checklists," reviews the isolation procedures in detail. Wearing the personal protective equipment (PPE) described is a type of isolation referred to as *contact isolation*.

> **EXAM ALERT**
>
> Remember the required sequence for donning and removing an isolation gown, gloves, and mask used in a contact isolation procedure. Review other precautions for specific clinical conditions as outlined in your facility procedure manual or your textbook.

Sharp Objects

Make every effort to avoid accidental needle sticks or cuts with sharp objects (often referred to as *sharps*).

Keep needles or sharp objects away from residents when not in use.

> **CAUTION**
>
> Be careful when changing resident linens, because they are a common site for discarded needles.

Promptly report to your supervisor any needle stick or puncture wound by a sharp object. You and other health-care workers are at high risk for transmission of *Hepatitis B (HBV)*, a blood-borne pathogen, or *human immunodeficiency virus (HIV)*. Infection with HIV can destroy the body's immune system and lead to other infections and AIDS. Infection caused by these viruses can result from a needle stick or other skin puncture by an instrument with contaminated blood on it.

> **CAUTION**
>
> Follow the procedure outlined in your facility's procedure manual regarding follow-up care and observation as directed for accidental exposure. Follow-up procedures in cases of accidental exposure to blood-borne pathogens is an example of *risk management* to help ensure resident and employee safety.

Care of residents with HIV infection, AIDS, and other special needs is discussed in Chapter 5, "Specialized Care."

> **CAUTION**
>
> If you must handle sharps containers, be careful not to force needles, syringes, or other sharp objects into the container. Close, seal, and dispose of sharps containers per agency protocol. To avoid accidental exposure as previously described, *never* empty sharp containers.

Resident Equipment

To ensure resident safety, adhere to facility policies regarding the use, care, and disposal of resident care equipment, because equipment used to care for residents can harbor pathogens that put them and you at risk.

▶ Clean and reprocess reusable equipment if used for multiple residents.

▶ Use equipment carefully to prevent exposure to resident blood and body fluids.

▶ Protect other residents from cross-contamination (spreading pathogens from one resident to another).

Environment

Follow facility policies and procedures to keep residents' environment as safe as possible, which includes keeping equipment, resident furniture, and personal articles free from contamination. Wipe spills from environmental surfaces promptly, disinfect them, and follow established procedures for removal of hazardous wastes, defined as any waste material that can cause infection. Hazardous wastes include any body fluids, such as blood.

EXAM ALERT

Remember those articles that must be discarded in a special biohazard container.

Linens

Keep resident linen from touching the floor; if it does, change it promptly. When soiled, remove linen immediately (fold the contaminated side inward and carry linen away from your body), tie the soiled linen inside a plastic bag, and deposit the bag in the facility's soiled linen area.

CAUTION

Dispose of dirty linen or other contaminated articles immediately. Do not wait for other team members to do so, because infection control is everyone's responsibility.

Surgical Asepsis

Surgical asepsis means using a sterile technique to protect against infection before, during, and after surgery by removing as many microorganisms as possible. When assisting the nurse with sterile procedures (for example, positioning the resident), avoid touching equipment or other objects placed in the sterile field. Touching such equipment or objects causes the treatment area to be contaminated.

Resident Safety

Residents have a right to feel safe and secure in the long-care environment. An important responsibility of a nursing assistant is to maintain their safety. Safety and security includes the following:

- **Protection from falls:** The most common accident for residents is a fall, often from a wet, slippery floor, or from equipment or supplies left in the resident's path, or by equipment that is damaged or improperly used. Watch constantly for environmental hazards that can place residents at risk for falls. This includes assuring adequate lighting of the residents' rooms; providing residents with reading glasses, canes, and other ambulation devices in good working order; removing spills and clutter in residents' environment; keeping frequently used supplies within easy reach of residents; assisting at-risk residents with ambulation; and keeping residents' beds in the lowest position. Restraints or other devices used to protect residents from harming themselves or others are discussed in Chapter 5.

- **Proper identification:** Mistakes in care can occur by failing to properly check residents' identification. Always check residents' armbands before serving their meals, performing nursing care, or other tasks that can place residents at risk.

- **Fire safety:** Protecting residents from fires is of utmost importance, because many residents cannot protect themselves, especially when a fire requires emergency evacuation. When a fire occurs, remember the R.A.C.E. system:

  - **R**emove all residents in the immediate area of the fire.

  - **A**ctivate the fire alarm and notify others of the fire.

  - **C**ontain the fire by closing all doors in the area of the fire.

  - **E**xtinguish the fire.

- Frequent fire drills using the facility's fire emergency plan is an important strategy to help prepare all personnel and the residents for a real fire emergency. Residents might also be evacuated in case of a bomb threat or other environmental crisis; follow the facility's evacuation plan for these situations as well.

- **Protection against abuse:** Residents' rights have been highlighted in Chapter 2, "The Roles and Responsibilities of the Nursing Assistant." Be alert for signs of abuse or neglect, and immediately report any suspicions you might have to your supervisor.

Reporting Accidents or Incidents

An incident report must be completed and filed with the facility's risk manager or other designated employee whether or not injuries resulted from an accident involving a resident. Incident reports serve to accurately record what occurred, when it occurred, and all details of the event, because problems related to the incident might occur sometime later. You must participate in filing the form if you were directly involved in the accident or witnessed it. Incident reports provide a record of the accident and offer valuable information leading to policy changes as needed to improve service to residents.

Exam Prep Questions

1. What is the second leading cause of death in an individual 65 years of age or older?

   - ○ **A.** Car accident
   - ○ **B.** Falls
   - ○ **C.** Choking
   - ○ **D.** Drowning

2. Which of the following is not an example of contamination caused by droplet transmission?

   - ○ **A.** Pneumonia
   - ○ **B.** Influenza
   - ○ **C.** Cold
   - ○ **D.** Hepatitis B

3. When equipment is used by multiple residents, it is important to decrease the opportunity for contamination. One way to avoid contamination is by cleaning the equipment with the cleanser provided by the institution. When should the equipment be cleansed?

   - ○ **A.** Before using the equipment again
   - ○ **B.** At the end of the shift
   - ○ **C.** After use by every resident
   - ○ **D.** At the time of each scheduled cleaning

4. The nursing assistant notices the smell of smoke as he passes by a resident's room. He enters the room and sees that a pillow is on fire in the empty bed next to where a resident is sleeping. What should be the nursing assistant's first action according to the RACE plan?

   - ○ **A.** Confine
   - ○ **B.** Alarm

    ○ **C.** Extinguish

    ○ **D.** Rescue

5. Which of the following is not considered appropriate handling of linen?

    ○ **A.** Changing it promptly when soiled

    ○ **B.** Folding the soiled portion inward

    ○ **C.** Depositing the soiled linen on the floor

    ○ **D.** Carrying the linen away from your body

6. Which of the following are age-related changes?

    ○ **A.** Decreased vision and hearing

    ○ **B.** Lower intelligence level

    ○ **C.** Difficulty communicating

    ○ **D.** Ability to learn a new skill

7. Which of the following actions is not a part of standard precautions?

    ○ **A.** Washing hands before and after contact with a resident

    ○ **B.** Wearing gown, goggles, and gloves whenever entering a resident's room

    ○ **C.** Wearing goggles when there is a possibility of splashes

    ○ **D.** Using gloves when there is a possibility of contact with body fluids

8. Before serving a resident a meal, it is important for the nursing assistant to properly check that the meal belongs to the resident by performing which of the following activities?

    ○ **A.** Checking the resident's identification according to facility policy.

    ○ **B.** Asking the roommate to identify the resident.

    ○ **C.** Asking the resident to identify self.

    ○ **D.** There is no need to check identification because you see the resident several times a week.

9. The registered nurse calls for your help to assist with a resident who has fallen on the floor. You know this incident must be reported to the risk manager of the facility. Which of the nurse's following actions would best relay the events that occurred?

    ○ **A.** Writing a note to the physician

    ○ **B.** Completing an incident report

    ○ **C.** Calling the director for the facility

    ○ **D.** Completing an adverse drug reaction form

10. A nursing assistant comes to work complaining of a sore throat, fever, and chills. She knows the unit is short a nursing assistant for today, so she did not call in sick. Which of the following is the best action of the nurse who is in charge?

   ○ **A.** Give the nursing assistant who is ill medication.

   ○ **B.** Allow the nursing assistant who is ill to rest after a.m. care is completed.

   ○ **C.** Instruct all the nursing assistants on the unit to work in pairs.

   ○ **D.** Send the ill nursing assistant home.

11. In the R.A.C.E. acronym, the C stands for

   ○ **A.** Collect

   ○ **B.** Call

   ○ **C.** Calm

   ○ **D.** Confine

12. Nursing assistants should always check residents' armbands before serving their meals, performing nursing care, or other tasks.

   ○ **A.** False

   ○ **B.** True

Answer Rationales

1. **B.** The second leading cause of death in the elderly is due to falls or complications resulting from falls. A car accident (A) is a safety issue that is sometimes overlooked in the elderly, but it is not a leading cause of death. Many elders have trouble swallowing due to an illness (C). Drowning (D) is not a leading cause of death in the elderly.

2. **D.** Hepatitis B is transmitted through blood that is contaminated with Hepatitis B. Pneumonia (A), Influenza (B), and the common cold (C) are all transmitted via respiratory droplets.

3. **C.** Equipment used for more than one resident is cleaned immediately after each use. Before using the equipment again (A) is incorrect because of the length of time that might occur between use from one resident to another. At the end of the shift (B) is incorrect because the nursing assistant on the next shift might not realize the equipment was not cleaned after it was used on the resident. At the time of each scheduled cleaning (D) is incorrect because scheduled cleaning is for regular deep cleaning of all equipment.

4. **D.** With RACE, the first action is to rescue any person who might be in danger from the fire. In this case, it is the resident sitting next to the empty bed. Confine (A), alarm (B), and extinguish (C) are all incorrect because they leave the resident in harm's way.

5. **C.** Depositing linen on the floor causes the soiled linen to contaminate the floor and become a hazard. Changing linen promptly when soiled (A), folding the soiled portion inward (B), and

carrying the linen away from your body (D) are a part of the procedure for the care of linen. When linen is soiled, it is promptly removed, and then the contaminated side is folded inward and carried away from your body to not contaminate the nursing assistant's uniform.

6. **A.** Decreased hearing and vision are age-related changes. Lower intelligence level (B) is incorrect because the loss of intellectual abilities as you get older is a myth. Difficulty communicating (C) is incorrect because most elders do not have problems with communicating unless they have suffered a stroke. The ability to learn a new skill is not impaired in the elderly (D).

7. **B.** Protective equipment is chosen according to the possible substance the health-care worker might have contact with. Washing hands before and after contact with a resident (A), wearing goggles when there is possibility of splashes (C), and using gloves when there is a possibility of contact with body fluids (D) are all part of standard precautions to protect the health-care worker.

8. **A.** It is important to follow facility policy of identifying residents. The most common way is by checking the resident's arm band; some facilities use pictures for identification. Asking the roommate to identify the resident (B), asking the resident to identify self (C), and not checking identification because you see the resident several times a week (D) are sometimes used along with choice A but not as the sole source of identification.

9. **B.** An incident report serves to accurately record what occurred, when it occurred, and all the details of the event because problems related to the incident might occur sometime later. Writing a note to the physician (A) is incorrect because the physician is called as soon as possible to update him or her on the condition of the resident. Calling the director of the facility (C) is wrong because the risk manager is responsible to investigate any accidents or incidents. Completing an adverse drug reaction form (D) is wrong because an adverse drug reaction form is completed only when an incident occurred due to a medication.

10. **D.** The best action of the nurse is to send the ill nursing assistant home to protect the other employees and the residents from spreading infection. Giving the nursing assistant who is ill medication (A), allowing the nursing assistant who is ill to rest after a.m. care is completed (B), and instructing all the nursing assistants on the unit to work in pairs (C) exposes others to illness, and those in a weakened state of health could contact the illness.

11. **D.** The first action if a fire occurs is to Rescue any person who might be in danger from the fire. The second step is to pull the Alarm or call for help. The C in the RACE stands for Confine. The last step is to Extinguish

12. **B.** The identity of residents is to be checked before serving their meals, performing nursing care, or any other tasks.

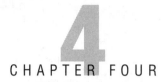

CHAPTER FOUR

Promotion of Function and Health of Residents

Medical Term Hotlist

Abduction	Contracture
Adduction	Convalescence
ADEs	Dangling
AM care	Defecate
Ambulation	Dehydration
Ambulation assistive device	Delirium
Analgesia	Dentition
Apical pulse	Dentures
Aspiration	Diastolic pressure
Atrophy	Dorsiflexion
Autonomy	Dysphagia
Axilla	Dyspnea
Blood pressure	Ecchymosis
Body alignment	Emesis
Body mechanics	Extension
Body temperature	Fecal impaction
Braden scale	Fever
Calorie	Flatus
Cerebral vascular accident (CVA)	Flexion
Coccyx	Fowler's position
Commode	Gait-transfer belt

Geri chair	Prone position
Graduate	Radial pulse
HS care	Range of motion (ROM)
Hydration	Rapport
Hygiene	Respirations
Hypertension	Restorative care
Immobilize	Rotation
Intake and output (I & O)	Self-actualization
Lateral position	Sim's position
Logroll	Stool
Malnutrition	Supination
Mechanical lift	Sphygmomanometer
Noncompliance	Stethoscope
NPO	Supine position
Nutrient	Syncopy
Oral hygiene	Systolic pressure
Perineal care	Tympanic membrane
PO	Urinate
Podiatry	Void
Pressure ulcer	

Nearly half of the written exam (WE) contains questions about your nursing skills. This chapter focuses on the key principles involved in providing resident care, organized into the following categories:

▶ Personal Care Skills

▶ Restorative Skills

▶ Psychosocial Skills

▶ Recording and Reporting

You must also review all skills as outlined in the performance checklists in Chapter 6, "Clinical Skills Performance Checklists." Critical steps for safe skills performance often reflect the key principles reviewed here; these critical steps must be met to successfully pass the Clinical Skills Test (CST), which tests your competencies in the following categories.

Personal Care Skills

The focus of this category is a review of direct care you provide residents on a daily basis to promote their health and well-being.

Activities of Daily Living

Assisting residents with activities of daily living (ADLs) is one of your primary responsibilities. The sections that follow describe the skills involved with ADLs.

Hygiene

It is important for residents to feel clean and fresh. Equally important is to keep the residents free from disease due to harmful bacteria that can enter the body through any skin break, which includes mucous membranes that line any body cavity. With aging, the skin produces less oil, which makes it dry, requiring less frequent bathing. This does not mean that a daily partial bath is not needed to freshen the mouth and *perineal* area (area of the body that includes the male and female genitalia and the anus). Cleanliness also removes body sweat, odors, and other secretions. Morning care (*AM care*) that includes washing the resident's face and hands followed by tooth brushing or denture care before eating breakfast helps decrease harmful bacteria, maintain a pleasant appearance, and increase a sense of well-being for the resident. Hygiene care before bedtime, often called *HS* (hour of sleep) *care*, accomplishes the same goals and promotes rest and sleep. HS care also might include a back rub or other form of massage to relax the resident.

Bathing

The resident's bath schedule as determined by the care plan might require a complete bath, shower, or a partial bath. Remember the general goals of skin care when bathing the resident; that is, to remove pathogens and promote comfort. Bathing promotes cleanliness, helps improve circulation by stimulating the muscles, provides exercise for the joints and limbs, and gives you the opportunity to inspect the resident's skin, mobility, and other signs of health and well-being. It also provides a time for personal interaction with residents that helps increase their self-esteem.

Safety, security, and privacy are key considerations with each type of bath. Allow the resident to participate in all aspects of personal care and grooming to promote self-control. Residents have taken care of themselves all of their lives and need to feel they can be independent as much as possible. Independence, decision making, and self-control are also known as having *autonomy*. Feeling secure is second only to being safe from harm. Protect residents from accidents while bathing, which includes falls, and from undue exposure due to failure to provide privacy during the bathing procedure. Posting privacy signs, using a privacy curtain, or closing the door, as well as shielding the body while bathing, are all essential steps to ensure privacy.

> **EXAM ALERT**
>
> For residents who are high risk for falls while bathing in the tub or shower, use an assistive device to help secure them in the shower chair or tub. Follow agency policy and accepted procedure when using any assistive device. Unauthorized use of these assistive devices could be considered a restraint.

Skin care involves keen observation of any breaks in the skin or other abnormalities that might indicate injury or disease. Keeping the skin moist but not wet, dry in the *axilla* (armpits) and *perineum*, and free from pressure are very important steps to protect the resident. Be sparing with lotions or other emollients for keeping skin supple. Avoid talcs, powders, or other products that can cake within skin folds. Areas, such as the *axilla*, beneath the breasts, the genitalia, buttocks, and other skin creases, are warm and moist, which can encourage bacterial growth.

> **EXAM ALERT**
>
> Only a licensed nurse can apply prescription ointments, lotions, or other products in any form to the skin; however, you are responsible for reporting any redness, pain, tenderness (signs of *inflammation*), open sore, or other skin abrasion immediately to the licensed nurse.

A skin break can result in a *pressure ulcer* (also called a bedsore, or *decubitus ulcer*) found over any bony part, such as the tailbone (*coccyx*), hip, back, elbow, breasts, spine, shoulder, or the back or side of the head. The term bedsore is misleading because a pressure ulcer can occur outside of bed by prolonged sitting or any pressure on the skin that decreases the blood supply to that area. Follow the facility's protocol for care of residents who are high risk, often evaluated according to the *Braden scale*, a guide used by the licensed nurse for describing the skin's risk for breakdown. Residents who are *immobile* (cannot move or walk), have a poor nutrition status, or have trouble healing are considered high risk for pressure ulcers and must be observed closely for any skin breakdown. Pressure ulcers are very painful and difficult to heal, leading to other complications and misery for the resident. The best approach to bedsores is prevention. Additional steps to prevent bedsores are incorporated into personal skills, such as positioning and turning the immobile resident, protecting bony prominences from undue pressure, using protective devices and equipment, and keeping the resident dry, comfortable, well nourished, and hydrated, as outlined in Chapter 5, "Specialized Care."

The following are other general principles that apply to bathing and grooming:

▶ Use standard precautions for personal care.

▶ Keep bathwater temperature at a safe level.

▶ Use mild soaps or other cleansers per facility policy, watching for resident allergies to bath products.

▶ When cleansing the body, wash from the cleanest area to the dirtiest area.

▶ For the complete bed bath, change water, wash cloth, and gloves prior to bathing the lower body and extremities.

▶ If assisting the resident to bathe, provide for rest so as not to overly tire the resident.

CAUTION

Be alert for residents who become weak, dizzy, or faint (*syncope*) during the bath, taking steps to protect them from falls or other accidents. If such a situation occurs, stop the bath process, stay with the resident, and call for assistance; report the incident to the licensed nurse immediately.

▶ Avoid touching the floor with bath towels, the remote shower spray head, or other bath equipment, because the floor is considered contaminated.

▶ Disinfect the tub, shower, and other bath articles following the bath or shower.

▶ Promptly remove soiled bath linens.

▶ Report and record the bath/grooming procedure and the resident's response.

Oral Care

Residents might need assistance with oral care, which can include brushing the resident's teeth or denture care. Dentures are false teeth, which might replace all or part of the resident's own teeth; they are necessary for proper eating, to retain the shape of the face, and to promote a positive self-image. With gloved hands, hold dentures over the sink to clean them. Pad the sink area with paper towels or a washcloth and water to provide safety against breakage in case the dentures are dropped during cleaning. Breaking dentures without taking those precautions can result in charges of negligence against you or the agency.

CAUTION

Do not use a regular toothbrush on dentures because the toothbrush will scratch the dentures, creating places for harmful bacteria to grow. Bacteria growth can cause mouth infections and bad breath.

With gloved hands, use a denture brush, a toothette, or washcloth to remove obvious particles on the dentures. Handle them gently, and wash and rinse them in warm (*tepid*) water to avoid damaging the dentures. Cover them with water and add an effervescent denture tablet to complete the cleaning process. After cleaning, store the dentures in a designated container labeled with the resident's name.

> **CAUTION**
>
> Take every precaution to prevent accidental loss of residents' dentures because this incident is costly, disposes the resident to nutritional problems, and is emotionally upsetting. Report lost dentures immediately.

In addition to teeth brushing, keep the mouth moist and free of debris. Dry mucous membranes in the mouth encourage bad breath and skin breakdown along with tooth decay. Depending on the resident's condition, you might need to provide oral care hourly or every two hours.

> **EXAM ALERT**
>
> When giving oral care to a comatose resident (one who is unconscious), turn the resident's head to the side and gently swab his or her mouth and mucous membranes with the recommended equipment and supplies while being careful not to cause the resident to aspirate, which means accidentally drawing food or fluid into the air passage.

Because the comatose resident breathes through the mouth, frequent oral care is needed to help clear secretions and keep the mouth and membranes well hydrated.

Grooming

Grooming includes hair care, shaving, nail care, and eyeglasses and hearing aid care. A resident who is well-groomed feels better and has a more positive outlook and self-esteem. Grooming principles mirror those for ADLs in general regarding standard precautions, providing privacy for the resident, and encouraging the resident to participate in ADLs as much as possible, which includes making choices that will increase satisfaction and compliance with the daily care plan. Remember to dress residents appropriately and comfortably in their own clothing. Consider weather and environmental changes for each resident; make clothing adjustments accordingly to maintain a comfortable body temperature. Because some residents might lose body fat, they can become chilled more easily, requiring a light wrap, sweater, or extra bed covering. Always check with the residents to determine their clothing and comfort needs.

Shaving

Shaving residents requires careful technique to avoid accidental nicking of the skin, which can create an entry for pathogens. Residents who have prolonged blood clotting for any reason might be required to shave with an electric razor. Check the resident's care plan for directions on how to manage his shaving needs.

Nail Care

Like skin care, nail care requires careful cleansing, frequently accomplished when washing the resident's hands. Keeping nails trimmed and clean can improve appearance while preventing injury or infection transmitted by dirty, unkempt nails. Soaking the resident's hands and feet in warm water helps loosen debris and eases nail trimming and cuticle care.

> **NOTE**
>
> In most states, CNAs may not trim resident's nails because of the possibility of exposing the resident to injury/infection. Risk for infection is especially related to residents with diabetes mellitus. If you assess that the resident's toenails need trimming, notify the nurse, who will make arrangements for a podiatry consult.

> **CAUTION**
>
> Dry between the resident's fingers and toes to prevent skin breakdown; avoid lotion between the fingers and toes to prevent bacterial growth.

Aging can cause the toenails to become thick and difficult to manage. Despite the need to keep nails trimmed, special consideration must be made for residents with diabetes because their toenails must be trimmed very carefully to avoid cuts on the foot that, due to poor circulation or diabetes, might not heal properly. Consult the facility's policy for nail care required for residents with special conditions such as diabetes. Refer to Chapter 5 for more information on foot care for the diabetic resident.

Hair Care   Clean hair that is neatly combed helps improve the self-image of residents and contributes to their general well-being. Each facility has a policy for hair care, including shampooing. In some facilities, shampooing the hair might require a doctor's order. Many residents might have their hair washed, set, and combed by a beautician who provides cosmetology services in the long-term care facility. Being sensitive to each resident's unique grooming needs is the hallmark of effective nursing assistant practice. Consult with the resident and family to learn the best approach for hair care, realizing that not all hair can be managed in the same way by different races or cultures. Consult with the licensed nurse when deciding the most effective approach.

Nutrition

Food is necessary for life. The fuel needed for adequate life functions comes from calories in food, defined as units of heat measurement. Caloric intake through foods gives the body the energy it needs. Elders, like younger adults, need the same kinds of nutrients, including vitamins and minerals. However, in the long-term care setting, residents must depend on caregivers for their nutritional needs. Although the diet of each resident must contain a balance of proteins for cell growth and healing, carbohydrates for ready energy, and fats for fueling the cells, the caloric needs of residents vary according to their activity level and their health status. Nutrition also includes fluid intake to maintain adequate hydration needed for all cellular functions in the body, especially digestion of foods. Fluid intake is required to replace losses through perspiration, respirations, evaporation, and normal elimination. Fluid intake also helps regulate body temperature as well as the moisture in the skin and mucous membrane. Aging can affect the sense of taste, smell, and thirst, which can cause a decrease in solid food and fluid intake. Other factors can affect resident nutrition, such as level of awareness, dentition, and the ability to chew properly; cultural considerations (religion, personal preferences, and family traditions); emotional well-being (depression, isolation, frustration, and anger); and the long-term care environment. If the resident's care plan specifies a special diet, the resident might not be satisfied with the diet and refuse to follow it. This is an example of noncompliance, meaning the resident does not adhere to the diet order. Noncompliance with diet can lead to malnutrition (inadequate consumption or absorption of food) or dehydration, meaning there is not enough fluid in the body that can cause serious problems in all body systems.

Edema, the opposite of dehydration, occurs when there is too much fluid in the body from excessive fluid intake or nutritional imbalances (such as too much salt or protein imbalance), certain medications, or disease processes. Edema, from accumulation of fluid in the body tissues, is often seen as swelling of the ankles, puffiness around the resident's eyes or all over the face, swelling of fingers, which causes rings to be excessively tight, or an increase in the diameter (roundness) of the abdomen. With edema, socks, sleeves, rings, or other clothing may leave a deep imprint on the skin where edema exists. Unless relieved, the local edema may decrease blood flow to the affected area, causing pain or inability to use the body part(s) affected.

CAUTION

Notify the nurse if a resident develops edema as previously described.

Remember these factors when assisting the resident with meals, fluids, and snacks to help maintain adequate nutritional status. The following guidelines can help achieve this goal:

▶ Diet permitting, offer the resident choices in the menu to encourage independence and sense of control.

▶ Make mealtime as pleasant an experience as possible. If the resident is dining in his or her room, remove noxious odors, bedpans, urinals, and anything that could negatively affect the resident's appetite. In the dining room, seat residents together who encourage pleasant social interaction.

▶ If the resident is dining alone, encourage social interaction, offering assistance as needed and conversation that helps increase resident satisfaction with the dining experience.

▶ Converse with the resident during the meal. Conversation, even when one-sided, helps to make the dining experience more pleasant.

▶ Present food as attractively as possible.

▶ Keep hot foods hot and cold foods cold.

▶ Offer fluids as often as possible according to the diet order.

▶ Assist with feeding as needed to encourage adequate nutrition.

EXAM ALERT

Review the feeding skills in Chapter 5, focusing on the critical steps to prevent choking and aspiration.

▶ Be patient with slow eaters and praise progress as needed to help increase motivation.

▶ Encourage physical activity to help improve the appetite.

▶ Individualize approaches to meals that recognize cultural needs—for example, offering a kosher diet, involving family or friends to assist with meals or feeding, praying before eating, and so on.

▶ If diet permits, encourage family members or friends to bring favorite foods from home or the community that appeal to the resident.

As with other nursing skills, accurately record and report all dietary intake, including fluids. Review the I & O skill in Chapter 6, "Clinical Skills Performance Checklists," for critical steps regarding charting meal consumption.

NOTE

Record I & O using the metric system or the measurement as specified in the I & O skill checklist in Chapter 6.

Toileting

Aging can affect the nervous system that controls elimination of body wastes like urine and feces (also known as *stool* or solid waste). The urge or need to *void*, or urinate (pass urine from the body) or *defecate* (pass feces from the body) decreases with age, often meaning that the resident is not aware of voiding or defecating until it actually happens. Decreased appetite and thirst, coupled with less food and fluid intake as well as slower digestion of foods, contribute to elimination problems. Infirmity or being unable to get to the toilet in time to avoid accidental soiling of clothing by urine or feces is not only potentially dangerous due to the increased risk of falls but also embarrassing for the resident.

Other factors might interfere with normal elimination, such as certain medications that could cause constipation or diarrhea, inactivity, pelvic muscle weakness due to aging, and nervous disorders. Small, watery leakage of stool could indicate a *fecal impaction*, a condition in which hard feces is trapped in the large intestine and rectum and cannot be pushed out by the resident. *Diarrhea*, on the other hand, results when food wastes pass too quickly through the intestine so that water is not reabsorbed adequately. This causes a watery brown liquid to be expelled, which leads to local skin irritation and a dangerous imbalance in the resident's fluid and electrolyte status. Both conditions require immediate reporting to the licensed nurse as well as prompt intervention to prevent further complications.

Remember the following principles when assisting the resident with toileting:

▶ Assisting the resident to void or defecate on a routine, timely basis to maintain normal elimination pattern and avoid accidents

▶ Being alert to individual toileting needs and prepare accordingly to help prevent accidents

▶ Observing standard precautions when handling urine or stool

▶ Using a bedpan, urinal, or bedside commode (portable toilet), and other procedures to maintain a normal elimination schedule

▶ Performing careful skin care following voiding or defecating

▶ Assisting the resident to wash his or her hands after toileting

▶ Observing, reporting, and recording excess or decreased output

Chapter 5 reviews guidelines for special care regarding elimination (for example, catheter care, ostomy care, enema procedure, and so on).

Rest, Sleep, and Comfort

Elders need as much sleep as other adults. Their ability to sleep might be influenced by the long-term care environment, especially when newly admitted, their activity level, their general state of health, and their individual habits. Naps or rest periods are essential for health and well-being and should be included in the resident's care plan. However, excessive napping during the day can interfere with sleep as well as signal a febrile illness or neurological complication. Residents might also awaken from sleep confused or *delirious*, meaning a state of agitated confusion. This situation is a sign of decreased oxygen to the brain that leads to the confusion. Report any change in *consciousness* (the awakened state), awareness or alertness, sleepiness for no obvious reason, and the inability to respond verbally.

Pain or discomfort can also interfere with rest and sleep. Pain might go unreported by the resident whose pain tolerance (ability to carry out activities or rest despite pain) is high or who has lost the ability to perceive pain. Likewise the resident might deny pain but act in other ways that indicate discomfort, which might include loss of appetite, refusal to participate in recreational activities, inability to sleep (*insomnia*), or withdrawing from social contact. Residents might also be less likely to report pain if they believe they will be labeled as complainers.

NOTE

Be careful to accept a resident's report of pain or discomfort at face value.

Physical signs of pain include increased pulse (*tachycardia*), increased respirations (*tachypnea*), difficulty breathing (*dyspnea*), and high blood pressure (*hypertension*). Sweating, crying, grunting, moaning, and other indicators of distress can indicate pain as well. The nurse can assess the resident's pain on a scale of 0–5 (zero meaning no pain to a score of five, which means it hurts enough to cry). The nurse might administer an analgesic, a drug to relieve pain. If the resident receives analgesia, you must assist the nurse in observing the resident's response to the medication, any dramatic change in the resident's vital signs after receiving the medication, and the resident's report of pain relief. Any abnormal reactions (known as *ADEs*, or adverse drug effects) to analgesia can include a sudden drop in blood pressure or respirations, dyspnea (rapid breathing), a rash on the body, and emotional distress. These signs require immediate intervention, so report them immediately to the nurse. Skills related to respiratory distress or cardiac emergencies are discussed in Chapter 5. You can assist the resident to rest more comfortably by changing the resident's position, offering diversion activities (reading, listening to music, meditation, and so on), providing a massage, and creating a quiet environment.

The following are general principles of care to promote rest and sleep:

► Maintaining the individual resident's routine to promote safety and security that encourages rest and sleep

► Arranging the resident's environment to decrease noise and confusion

► Pacing resident activities to arrange for rest periods during the day and an effective sleep schedule

► Using positioning devices to increase comfort

► Offering emotional support when the resident is experiencing pain and discomfort

► Promoting safety by keeping the bed in the lowest position; locking the wheelchair when the resident is sitting; keeping the urinal, bedpan, or bedside commode near the bed; and keeping a night light on for the resident when visiting the restroom during the night

▶ Arranging care routines to encourage rest; for example, spacing ADLs, recreational activities, and visiting times

▶ Refraining from judging the resident who reports pain. Residents may be less likely to report pain if they believe they will be labeled as complainers.

▶ Teaching the resident to avoid caffeine-free beverages at least three to four hours prior to bedtime, because caffeine acts as a stimulant, which promotes wakefulness.

Restorative Skills

Prevention is one of the most important approaches you use with residents. The steps you take to help prevent complications of immobility, for example, are critical for the resident. Other skills you perform include observing changes in the resident's status and reporting your findings so that immediate interventions can be made to ward off infection or infirmity. Restorative skills are those nursing duties you perform to help the resident function as normally as possible that goes beyond rehabilitation, a process of therapeutic treatments or approaches to restore and maintain the highest possible level of functioning a resident can possess. For example, physical therapists might assist the resident to walk, but the resident chooses to sit in a wheelchair all day and not ambulate, even though he or she is able; refusing to ambulate can result in a setback in his or her rehabilitation progress. Your encouragement and assistance to help motivate the resident to walk is preventive in nature because you are committed to maintaining the resident's restored function. It is also considered restorative because it involves more than physical therapy but emotional and psychological support. Feeding, assisting with toileting, and turning immobile residents are examples of preventive measures you take every day to prevent complications that can occur from inactivity, failure to maintain adequate nutrition, and skin breakdown from toileting problems.

Self-Care and Independence

The Omnibus Budget and Reconciliation Act (*OBRA*) of 1987 requires all long-term facilities to use every resource to help residents reach or maintain their highest level of physical, psychological, and mental functioning. The act requires that all residents have a right to make as many choices about their lives, their care, and their life style routines as possible. It is not only a legal requirement determined by OBRA but an ethical principle as well. Care guidelines discussed thus far have included self-care and independence. Adhering to residents' rights helps meet the letter of the law as well as the spirit of the law; that is, to protect residents' rights of a comfortable and caring environment in which they can live as safely and happily as possible.

> **NOTE**
>
> Unless their self-care decisions are dangerous to themselves or others, residents should be allowed and encouraged to make them.

The principles covered in the sections that follow apply to restorative skills.

Mobility/Immobility

Mobility is being able to move by one's self, to walk, and to exercise to help maintain muscle function and improve a sense of independence and self-worth. Moving, ambulating, and exercising help improve blood circulation and proper musculoskeletal functioning. *Immobility*, the opposite of being mobile, affects the total well-being of the resident; that is, by exposing the resident to alterations in almost every body system:

- ▶ In the circulatory system, an increased risk of blood clots (*thrombi*) and edema in the lower extremities, causing undue stress on the heart.

- ▶ Respiratory complications such as pneumonia, other infections of the respiratory tree, or failure to expand the lungs.

- ▶ In the digestive system, *anorexia*, or decreased appetite, and constipation.

- ▶ The musculoskeletal system suffers due to loss of calcium in the bones (called osteopenia), *atrophy*, or muscle wasting and *contractures* (deformities of the limbs due to immobility). The inability to walk also adds to an increased thinning and weakening of the bones, leading to osteoporosis, a chronic condition putting the resident at risk for fractures.

- ▶ Pressure ulcers on the skin.

Mentally and emotionally, the immobile resident might feel frustrated, isolated, depressed, and hopeless due to loss of autonomy and the need to rely on others. Socially, the resident loses self-esteem, has poor body image, and feels separated from social interaction.

Assisting the resident to maintain normal functional movement might include range of motion (*ROM*), which means freely moving all limbs and joints. If the resident cannot perform range of motion independently, you must perform passive range of motion exercises (*PROM*), which move the joints to protect the muscles from atrophy, increase circulation, and joint motion.

> **CAUTION**
>
> Follow the care plan instructions for PROM as well as the facility's policy for exercising the neck. Remember to avoid pushing the joint past the point of resistance or the point where pain occurs.

Range of motion includes *abduction* (moving the extremity away from the body), *adduction* (moving the extremity toward the body), *flexion* (bending the extremity), and *extension* (opposite of flexion). Report and record the PROM procedure and the resident's response to the exercises. Physical therapists or massage therapists might also provide exercises for the residents as part of the rehabilitation plan. Your care helps to restore the resident to normal functioning and support the plan.

When you assist the immobile resident with lifting, moving, or transferring, remember to:

▶ Use proper body mechanics.

▶ Explain what you are going to do.

▶ Ask for the resident's help as much as possible.

▶ Face the resident.

▶ Place your feet apart in line with your shoulders.

▶ Bend your knees.

▶ Keep your back straight.

▶ Reach close to the resident, protecting your balance, posture, and internal girdle (contract abdominal muscles and buttocks to protect the spine).

▶ Use both hands when lifting.

▶ Avoid twisting at the waist.

▶ When moving the resident's entire body, move the top first, the middle (torso) second, and then the legs; in certain situations, *logrolling* might be necessary, which is moving the body from side to side as one unit.

▶ Ask for assistance from another nursing assistant as needed to keep you and the resident safe.

▶ Use a mechanical lift, lift sheet, or other device as needed to promote safe lifting.

Positioning the immobile resident requires using the previous principles to keep the body in proper alignment. For immobile residents, use positioning devices (hand rolls, wedges, splints, shoes, or boots) to provide *dorsiflexion* (pointing toes of the foot toward the knee) and to prevent contractures, pressure ulcers, and discomfort. Review body positioning—for example, prone, supine, Sim's position, and Fowler's position, as well as using a mechanical lift discussed in Chapter 6.

EXAM ALERT

Critical steps in these procedures will most likely be included on the WE.

Transferring, or moving the resident from bed to chair, from bed to wheelchair, and from bed to stretcher requires proper body mechanics and the use of a *gait belt* or other assistance to prevent falling. Assisting the resident to walk is another important skill involved in ADLs. These skills are outlined in Chapter 6.

> **EXAM ALERT**
>
> **Proper body mechanics is of utmost importance to protect yourself and the residents when lifting, moving, transferring, and ambulating residents.**

Health Maintenance and Restoration

Health maintenance and restoration includes measuring vital signs, height, and weight. Vital signs include the temperature, pulse, respiration, and blood pressure—all essential elements of life; thus the term *vital*. Accurate measurement and recording are important skills in determining the overall health of the resident.

Careful attention to vital signs can save a life. Age-related factors that affect vital signs include age, sex, time of day in which vital signs are measured, illness, emotions, activity and exercise, food intake, and medications. Often, a change in one vital sign will affect the other vital signs. For example, when the resident has a fever (temperature over 101 degrees), the pulse rate and respirations will also increase.

It is important to weigh residents carefully as ordered. Consider clothing, shoes, and other articles when weighing the resident because weight can be affected by clothing. Report any dramatic changes in weight because these changes might indicate a nutritional deficiency, fluid retention, or a serious illness.

Determining resident height is an important measure when admitting a resident; record subsequent measurements at least annually or as required by facility protocols. Changes in posture due to problems in the musculoskeletal system can be determined by monitoring resident height.

General guidelines that apply to measuring vital signs are as follows:

▶ Explain the procedure to the resident.

▶ Delay measuring the oral (PO) temperature at least 15 minutes for residents who have recently smoked or who have had a hot liquid.

▶ Arrange the steps of measuring vital signs, height, and weight to conserve energy and increase efficiency.

EXAM ALERT

Follow product guidelines for use of tympanic thermometers, sphygmomanometers (blood pressure cuff), and stethoscopes to ensure accuracy in vital signs measurement.

▶ If taking an axillary temperature, make sure the axilla is dry; record the reading with an *A*, indicating the method used; and follow other facility guidelines for use of approved medical abbreviations or terms.

▶ If unsure of any reading, repeat the procedure and report your findings.

NOTE

Blood pressure measurements should be taken in the arm that records the highest reading with the resident sitting or lying. The initial blood pressure reading should be taken in both arms with the resident lying supine, sitting, and standing; record each measurement. Remember, when the resident is sitting, both feet should be flat on the floor. Do NOT take blood pressure in an arm if

▶ The arm is on the same side as a mastectomy.

▶ The arm has been affected by stroke or other debilitating injury or is malformed.

▶ The arm has a current IV infusion or a shunt in it.

▶ The radial pulse (pulse felt at the wrist) should be measured for at least one minute if the resident has heart disease. When taking the apical pulse (listening to the heartbeat at the apex, or tip of the heart), listen for at least one minute and record the reading. Review the apical-radial pulse procedure in Chapter 6. Report an irregular pulse (heartbeat), because the resident might be experiencing an abnormal heart condition.

▶ Respirations (includes inspiration and expiration) should be counted for one minute, noting any difficulty in breathing (dyspnea) or pauses in the rhythm of the respirations or the pulse.

▶ Review the facility's procedure for using a wheelchair scale or other equipment for immobile residents who cannot stand on a scale.

▶ Record and report vital signs, height, and weight promptly.

TIP

Carry a small pad or other means of recording the vital signs at the bedside so you will remember them; this is especially important when completing vital signs for multiple residents.

▶ Clean all vital sign equipment after each use, especially stethoscope heads, to prevent cross-contamination.

Psychosocial Care Skills

Assisting residents to meet their basic needs includes their emotional and mental well-being, also called *psychosocial needs*. These needs are as important as the physiological needs discussed previously. All residents living in a long-term care facility are no different from other people who need to feel worthwhile, loved, and secure in their relationships with others. Having these needs at least partially met can contribute to their overall health and welfare.

Emotional and Mental Health Needs

Being mentally and emotionally healthy means being able to cope with the effects of aging, adjusting to life changes such as being dependent on others, losing loved ones and friends, as well as changes in social life. Those who feel good about the past will often cope well with aging, remaining hopeful, and optimistic about the future. Adjusting to aging is a difficult time for some residents who might long for those more productive years, who have lost a spouse or significant other, and who must now face the future alone and in a strange environment. Memories for them might be painful, especially if they did not achieve their life goals or if they regret past experiences. Leaving the familiar surroundings of home, past friendships, and past lifestyle can be depressing for the resident who feels lonely and isolated. Equally, residents might also become depressed in the long-term care environment and feel resentment toward family who, in their opinion, abandoned them. Elders, especially widows and widowers, are at high risk for suicide because they can fall deeper and deeper into depression that might go unnoticed by family, friends, or caregivers.

Caring about residents as well as for them is a key ethical component of nursing assistant practice. It is often easier to meet the physical needs of residents than to address their psychosocial and emotional needs. Actions, however, speak louder than words, such as spending time with residents, listening to them, showing interest in them and their lives, and encouraging social interaction with others. Being kind, considerate, and compassionate are attributes described in Chapter 1, "What You Need to Know to Prepare for the Exam"; they bear repeating here as well. Demonstrate your genuine concern and acknowledgement of each resident as a worthwhile person who deserves your respect and positive regard. Remember that, despite regional influences, you must always address residents by title and name, not "Grandma," "Mamma," "Honey," "Sweetie," or other forms of address that may be perceived by the resident as disrespectful and/or demeaning. When residents request to be called by their first name, add Mr., Mrs., or Miss to the first name to show respect.

You can encourage residents to participate in their care and activities, which will help improve their sense of independence, self-control, mood, and outlook. Encouraging family members and friends to visit and involving residents in activities helps to meet their social needs. Being observant when working with residents by watching and listening for cues to their mood is very important because you will spend more time with them than any other caregiver. Report any signs or symptoms of depression to the nurse so that interventions can be made to protect the resident and improve his or her quality of life in the long-term care facility.

Cultural Needs

Be aware of residents' unique needs, desires, and meaning in life based on their cultural practices. This is particularly important when planning care for residents that will satisfy them and build their trust. Table 4.1 is a review of views on health, illness, and caring by various cultural groups that might influence how you approach their care.

TABLE 4.1   Cultural Views of Health and Illness

	Western Cultures	Non-Western Cultures
Illness Causes	Biological or medical sources (germs, viruses, bacteria, body system malfunctions, and cancers)	Supernatural Religious Magical Supernatural
Illness Diagnosis	Scientific, system-specific pathology, use of technology	Naturalistic Holistic
Treatment of Illness by Practitioners/Healers	Medicine Surgery Educated according to established standards and qualifications for practice	Herbal Supernatural Magical/religious practices Learned through apprenticeship Reputation in the community as healer
Responsibility for Health or Illness	Self	Care provided by others; Rely on cultural group

Residents' cultural beliefs affect how they view illness or infirmity and, more importantly, how they respond to health problems. For example, people from certain non-western cultures believe that seizures result from the wandering of the soul, a supernatural cause. They might seek treatment from a shaman, or community healer who can perform a ritual to restore their soul. This is different from western cultural beliefs in the scientific explanation of seizures as being caused by a neurological abnormality. This cultural conflict could impact the resident's acceptance of traditional medication to treat a seizure.

Another example of cultural differences is the value in North American society in individualism, or the ability to take care of self and remain independent of others. Asians, Africans, and

Hispanics, however, rely on active family and community support and involvement in their care. This might be seen, for example, in an Asian elder who refuses rehabilitative care after hip surgery until her family can be present.

Many Southeast Asians use folk remedies, and Haitians and South Americans might use herbals, or potions, and wear jewelry (amulets) to ward off evil spirits that cause illness. Native Americans use prayers, chanting, and herbs to treat illness, often thought to stem from supernatural as well as physical causes.

Certain cultures also respond differently to pain and suffering. Asians might become stoic and choose not to report pain, whereas Hispanics might complain quite vocally when distressed.

These are only a few examples of how cultural differences of residents might affect their health and illness behavior. You must be able to understand each resident in light of his or her culture, being careful not to dismiss his or her beliefs or minimize the role that culture plays in health and well-being. Accepting cultural differences demonstrates your ability to truly accept all residents with dignity and care.

Spiritual Needs

Spirituality is defined as finding the inner meaning, or essence of life. Spiritual health refers to the wholeness of a person and the ability to connect with something larger than self. This sense of completeness or self-fulfillment is called *self-actualization* and, according to psychology, meets the highest level of basic human needs. Spirituality might be expressed by residents who find meaning in nature, music, or other expressions that reflect their beliefs of a supreme being or higher power. Healthy people have a positive spirit, meaning they find hope and confidence in the future. They view life with a sense of humor. The human spirit is also a powerful force when a person faces difficulties or life crises. The opposite of spiritual health in this case is called *spiritual distress*, or the feeling that the future is hopeless. Spiritual distress can lead to or increase the severity of illness or infirmity. Research describes elders who lose the will to live due to spiritual distress and, despite interventions to the contrary, die soon after hopelessness occurs.

Spirituality is often linked with an organized, formal religion that includes rituals and other behaviors that express faith; however, spirituality is not directly connected to religion. The freedom and opportunity to observe religious practices enables the resident to meet his or her spiritual needs and, thus, is important to maintain.

The best way to support resident's spiritual needs is to find out what matters most to them. Listen to what they say about spirituality and their spiritual needs. Establishing a caring relationship with residents, known as *rapport*, will help residents more openly talk about their spiritual needs and how you can support them. The following principles apply when addressing residents' spiritual needs:

▶ Organize care to enable residents the opportunity to practice their own religion.

▶ Handle any religious objects used by the resident with care and respect.

EXAM ALERT

Praying with residents or participating in their religious practices is appropriate but not required.

▶ If you are uncomfortable with participating in the resident's religious practices, consult with the licensed nurse who can refer the resident to a religious counselor or volunteer to assist with making religious services or other forms of spiritual expression possible.

▶ Stay open to residents whose beliefs and spiritual practices might differ from your own.

▶ Be careful not to ignore, disapprove of, or judge a resident's spiritual practices.

EXAM ALERT

Do not impose your own religious beliefs on residents. This is a form of prejudice, which is unacceptable in a health-care environment.

▶ Respect the resident's choice not to participate in religious activities.

▶ Encourage residents to express other forms of spirituality that do not include religious activities.

▶ Express your own spirituality to impart hope and a sense of humor when relating to residents.

Sexual Needs

Sexuality or expressing one's sexual needs for intimacy is important to residents and should not be ignored. Physical sexual expression involves more than lovemaking and includes touching, caressing, cuddling, and other forms of human touch. Psychologically, love and affection and a sense of belonging also involve sexual expression. Contrary to popular belief, sexual desire does not decrease with aging. However, the physical response to desire can be affected by neurological and circulatory changes due to conditions such as diabetes, cardiovascular disease, or chronic illness. It is important for you to be aware of your own feelings about sexuality to help residents meet their sexual needs.

Equally important is your knowledge that residents have a right to express their sexual feelings and must be given such opportunities as are appropriate in the long-term care setting. It is important to provide privacy for residents who need to express their sexual desires. Displays of affection toward you or other residents are normal according to the customs of common courtesy and social etiquette. However, you must frankly and clearly confront sexual behavior that is unacceptable to you or others. For example, if a resident makes unwanted sexual advances toward you or another resident, firmly and specifically state your objection to the advance. The resident may also refer to you as a "girlfriend" or "boyfriend," which is also unacceptable and presents an opportunity for misunderstanding should you tolerate the reference. Other unwelcome behavior may include flirting, which the resident might defend as merely teasing. Such defense is unacceptable, even if prompted or aided by illness, medication, or mental state. Kindly inform the resident that the behavior must stop immediately. Be as specific as possible, for example, "I need you to remove your hand from my breast immediately." Serious breaches of etiquette related to sexuality should be reported immediately to your supervisor in order to protect yourself and other residents.

Data Collection and Reporting

Your ability to observe residents while caring for them is an essential skill you bring to work. Collecting data and reporting changes in residents' conditions can be life saving. You spend the majority of your shift providing direct care to residents, which is a good time to learn from them what is happening to them and how they are progressing with their plan of care. Small changes in condition can make a big difference in a resident's well-being. For example, noticing a resident not talking with you as much as the day before might signal a developing infection or change in neurological status or mood. Changes in vital signs that might not seem alarming to others might alert you that the resident needs further assessment by the nurse. Assisting the resident with ADLs gives you the opportunity to use your sense of smell, touch, sight, and hearing to detect changes in the resident that warrant follow up. Using your senses helps validate what you can directly observe, also known as *objective assessment*. Subjective findings are those observations you conclude from what the resident reports to you that cannot be seen directly; these are also referred to as *symptoms*. Resident's statements of pain, distress, or general health belong to this category of observation and can be as significant as your direct observations. Be careful not to underestimate subjective reporting; take the resident's report at face value. Ignoring the resident's statements can cause you to miss important clues to health changes that could become life threatening if left unattended.

> **NOTE**
>
> *Following your gut*, which means your intuition or hunch, is actually based on past experience with residents and can serve you well in your work to keep residents safe and secure; don't ignore your intuition, but act on it.

General guidelines for data collection and reporting resident health status are as follows:

▶ When reporting changes in a resident's condition, use his or her own words as much as possible to promote objectivity and accuracy.

▶ Ask the resident to repeat any statements regarding his or her condition to be sure you understand what is being reported to you.

▶ Report any change in

   ▶ Vital signs, including weight changes

   ▶ Skin changes, including, but not limited to, cyanosis (blue skin color); size or appearance of moles or other skin lesions; skin temperature; and rashes or redness

   ▶ Weakness or dizziness; syncope (fainting)

   ▶ Signs or symptoms of abuse or neglect

   ▶ Edema anywhere in the body

   ▶ Mood changes or any change in resident behavior

   ▶ Coughing or spitting up blood

   ▶ Vomiting

   ▶ Diarrhea or constipation

   ▶ Environmental hazards

   ▶ Any suspicions that cannot be verified but that still cause you to feel concern for the resident's welfare

Recording resident information is another important task you perform daily. Recent changes in technology now might require a basic ability to use the computer or other electronic devices for documenting/recording care and observations. It is important to use correct grammar and spelling as well as acceptable medical terms and abbreviations.

EXAM ALERT

Review medical terms and abbreviations on the Cram Sheet to help you prepare for the WE.

If recording your observations and care on a written form, be sure to document in blue or black ink only and print legibly, accurately, and completely to ensure proper documentation of what occurred while working your shift. Sign your name and title to all entries. Record your work promptly to ensure accuracy and completeness; make corrections as needed according to the facility's guidelines. Never erase, scratch out, or use a liquid eraser to correct your charting.

If you record in error, strike it out with one line and your initials. Do not leave empty spaces. Remember that the resident's chart is a medical record and, as such, is a legal document and can be used in court.

TIP

Always record your work as though an attorney is reading it.

Be objective and descriptive in recording; never record your opinion. For example, when describing a reddened area on the heel of a resident, describe the size of the area (1×1-inch; dime-sized), color, whether the area is at or above the level of the skin and whether the area is warm to the touch. Refrain from stating your opinion as to why it is reddened, such as "the area is red because the last shift did not turn the resident." Expressing your opinion is not only opinion, it may jeopardize the agency by stating an observation with an opinion that implies negligence. You may, however, use resident direct quotes, but be careful to use quotation marks and not your interpretation of what the resident said.

Seek help from the nurse or your supervisor in charting situations that require consultation to ensure that your documentation is thorough, concise, and as objective as possible.

Exam Prep Questions

1. What are two general goals for a.m. care?

    ○ **A.** Remove soil and promote an increase in skin moisture.

    ○ **B.** Promote relaxation of the resident and decrease need for mobility.

    ○ **C.** Increase circulation and decrease incidence of pressure ulcers.

    ○ **D.** Remove harmful bacteria and promote well-being.

2. The nurse hands the nurse assistant a tube of medication and asks her to apply it after she has completed the resident's bath. Which of the following would be the nursing assistant's best response?

    ○ **A.** "I will gladly apply the medication as soon as I dry the skin."

    ○ **B.** "I don't have the time to do your job and mine too."

    ○ **C.** "As a nursing assistant, I can't apply medication without a nurse present in the room."

    ○ **D.** "As a nursing assistant, applying medication is beyond my scope of practice."

3. Which statement about taking an oral temperature is false?

○ **A.** The thermometer is placed in the mouth under the tongue in the sublingual pocket.

○ **B.** Wait 10 minutes if the resident has consumed any hot or cold liquids.

○ **C.** The normal oral temperature is 96.6°F.

○ **D.** Thermometer covers are used on all residents.

4. When should an apical pulse rate be repeated?

○ **A.** A pulse rate of 84 beats per minute

○ **B.** A pulse rate of 54 beats per minute

○ **C.** A pulse rate of 76 beats per minute

○ **D.** A pulse rate of 66 beats per minute

5. Which of the following definitions is true?

○ **A.** Tachycardia is a slow heart rate.

○ **B.** An irregular heart rate should be taken for at least 30 seconds.

○ **C.** The carotid site is used most often to obtain the pulse.

○ **D.** Bradycardia is a slow heart rate.

6. Which blood pressure should the nursing assistant repeat before reporting it to the nurse?

○ **A.** 90/60 mm Hg

○ **B.** 120/74 mm Hg

○ **C.** 140/68 mm Hg

○ **D.** 130/70 mm Hg

7. All of the following steps are part of the procedure for weighing residents, except what?

○ **A.** Residents are to remove shoes before weighing.

○ **B.** Residents are to void before being weighed.

○ **C.** Weights are obtained when the nursing assistant has time in the day's schedule.

○ **D.** Scales are to be calibrated to zero each day or routinely.

8. A resident who was very talkative earlier in the day is now difficult to awaken for his bath. The most appropriate action for the nursing assistant is which of the following?

○ **A.** Ask another nursing assistant if this has ever happened before.

○ **B.** Report the change in condition to the charge nurse immediately.

○ **C.** Realize he does not want his bath now and come back later.

○ **D.** Reposition the resident and make sure he is comfortable.

9. The nurse assistant might expect to find pressure ulcers in all of the following locations except where?

◯ **A.** Heels

◯ **B.** Nose

◯ **C.** Elbows

◯ **D.** Knees

10. Which of the following is false regarding assisting a resident with his or her bath?

◯ **A.** Have the room free from drafts.

◯ **B.** Assure the resident's privacy.

◯ **C.** Warm the bath water to between 110 and 115 degrees.

◯ **D.** Use only one washcloth and towel.

11. According to psychology, the highest basic need a person is able to obtain to promote health and well-being is

◯ **A.** Cultural needs

◯ **B.** Physical needs

◯ **C.** Sexual needs

◯ **D.** Spiritual needs

12. The CNA should always be instructed on equipment before using it.

◯ **A.** True

◯ **B.** False

Answer Rationales

1. **D.** The two primary goals of bathing are protection from harmful bacteria and promoting the well-being of the residents. Removing soil and promoting an increase in skin moisture (A) is incorrect because bathing might increase skin dryness, not decrease it. Promoting relaxation of the resident and decreasing need for mobility (B) is incorrect because residents require mobility to decrease morbidity. Increasing circulation and decreasing incidence of pressure ulcers (C) is incorrect because pressure ulcers are decreased by cleanliness and frequent change of position along with proper nutrition.

2. **D.** Nursing assistants are not to apply medications because they do not have a license, training, or knowledge to administer medications. The statements in choices A and C are incorrect because the nursing assistant is planning to administer the medication, which is not part of his or her role. The statement in choice B is incorrect due to the use of improper communication.

3. **C.** Normal oral temperatures are between 96.8°F and 100.4°F. Placing the thermometer in the mouth under the tongue in the sublingual pocket (A), waiting 10 minutes if the resident has consumed any hot or cold liquids (B), and using thermometer covers on all residents (D) are all steps used to determine the oral temperature.

4. **B.** The normal adult heart rate is between 60 to 100 beats per minute. A pulse rate of 84 (A), 76 (C), and 66 (D) are within the normal range.

5. **D.** Bradycardia is the heart rate below 60 beats per minute. Answer A, "Tachycardia is a slow heart rate," is incorrect; tachycardia is the heart rate above 100 beats per minute. Answer B, "An irregular heart rate should be taken for at least 30 seconds," is incorrect because irregular heart rates are to be obtained for one full minute. Answer C, "The carotid site is used most often to obtain the pulse," is incorrect; the radial site is used most often to obtain a resident's pulse.

6. **A.** Normal blood pressure for an adult is less than 120/80 and pre-hypertensive is less than 139/89. The blood pressure readings of 120/74 mm Hg, 140/68 mm Hg, and 130/70 mm Hg in choices B, C, and D are within normal limits.

7. **C.** Residents should be weighed at approximately the same time each day. Having the resident remove shoes (A), voiding (B) before being weighed, and calibrating the scales to zero each day or routinely (D) are part of the procedure for assuring accurate weighing of the residents.

8. **B.** Change in a resident's condition is serious and should be communicated to the nurse immediately. Answer A is not correct because assessment of the resident is not part of the nursing assistant's role. Answer C involves assumptions that might lead to harm of the resident. Answer D is incorrect because the first and most important action of the nursing assistant in this situation is to communicate immediately to the nurse the change in the resident's condition.

9. **B.** Pressure ulcers are more prone to develop in bony areas. The heels (A), elbows (C), and knees (D) are areas with the highest incidence of pressure ulcers, which are located on bony surfaces.

10. **D.** At least two washcloths and towels will be needed. One is for clean areas and the other for areas considered dirty. This is done to prevent spread of organisms. Keeping the room free from drafts (A), assuring the resident's privacy (B), and warming the bath water to between 110 and 115 degrees (C) are correct. The room is to be free of drafts, and the room temperature should be between 68°F and 74°F to prevent chilling. The resident's privacy is to be maintained at all times. Bath water temperature should be warm to promote comfort, help relaxation of muscles, and prevent chilling but should not be hot, which risks injury to the resident.

11. **D.** This sense of completeness or self-fulfillment is called and, according to psychology, meets the highest level of basic human needs. Answers A, B, and C are basic spiritual needs and are important to a patient's well-being; these needs must be met first before a person can reach the highest need of spirituality.

12. **A**. True. To operate any equipment, the CNA should first be instructed on the correct use so as not to harm the patient or themselves.

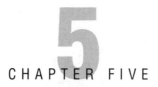

CHAPTER FIVE

Specialized Care

Medical Term Hotlist

Advance directive	Disoriented
AIDS	DNR
Alzheimer's disease	Dyspnea
AMI	Dysuria
Angina	Edema
Arteriosclerotic	Emaciated
Aphasia	Embolus
Carbohydrates	Emesis
Cardiac arrest	End of Life Issues
Cheyne-Stokes respirations	Enteral nutrition
Chronic illness	Euthanasia
Colostomy	Flaccid
Comatose	G tube
Congestive heart failure	Grief process
Coronary arteries	Hallucination
CPR	Hemiplegia
CVA	Hemorrhage
Cyanosis	Holistic health care
Debilitated	Hospice
Delusion	Hyperglycemia
Dementia	Hypertension
Diabetes	Hypoglycemia

Hypotension	Quadriplegia
Hypoxia	Reality orientation
Incontinence	Rescue breathing
Infusion-IV therapy	Respiratory arrest
Intubation	Respite care
Ketones	Restraint
KS	Role reversal
Malnutrition	Seizure
Mechanical ventilator	Sensory overload
Metastasis	Sensory stimulation
Nares	Sexually transmitted disease/illness (STD/STI)
Nocturia	Shroud
NPO	Sputum
Opportunistic disease	Stoma
Oxygen	Suffocation
Palliative care	Suicidal ideation
Paralysis	Sundowner's Syndrome
Paraplegia	Terminal illness
Patient Self Determination Act (PSDA)	Thrombus
PCP (Pneumocystis Carinii Pneumonia)	TIA
Plaque	TPN
Polyuria	Tracheostomy
Postmortem care	Tuberculosis (TB)
Postoperative	
Prosthesis	

This chapter reviews specialized care for residents experiencing more severe physical problems and psychological issues, and those who are dying. The skills involved in specialized care of these residents are discussed in Chapter 6, "Clinical Skills Performance Checklists."

Physical Problems

Physical problems reviewed in this section focus on acute and chronic conditions affecting major body systems.

Vision Impairment

Residents with hearing and vision problems are at high risk for injury, communication difficulties, and a potential for social isolation and loss of self-esteem. Common vision problems include chronic conditions such as glaucoma, a disease in which excessive pressure builds inside the eye that can cause blindness if left untreated. Cataracts, a clouding of the lens, prevents clear vision. Macular degeneration causes the loss of central vision while leaving side-to-side, or peripheral, vision intact. Diabetic retinopathy, a complication of diabetes, causes hardening of the arteries that carry blood and oxygen to the eye as well as damaging the retina. To ensure safety and security as well as improve their quality of life, it is important to assist residents with impaired vision by following these principles:

- ▶ Knock before entering the resident's room, identify yourself, and announce your entry.

- ▶ Keep the resident informed of the placement of room furniture and belongings.

- ▶ Arrange personal articles and other equipment and supplies within easy reach of the resident and encourage their use.

- ▶ Keep the resident's room clean, uncluttered, and safe.

- ▶ Maintain adequate lighting.

- ▶ To reduce glare, keep light sources behind the resident instead of behind you.

- ▶ Maintain the resident's bed in its lowest position.

- ▶ Explain everything you are about to do for the resident, and alert the resident when you have completed each task.

- ▶ Explain any extraordinary sounds in the environment.

- ▶ Stay within the resident's field of vision to enable the resident to focus on your face and voice.

- ▶ Speak in a pleasant tone of voice.

- ▶ Use a gentle touch to communicate.

- ▶ When assisting the visually impaired resident to eat, open cartons or assist with feeding but encourage as much independence with eating as possible.

- ▶ Use the hands of the clock to teach the resident the location of the foods on the plate.

- ▶ Ensure that the resident can locate and touch the light before leaving the room.

EXAM ALERT

If feeding a vision-impaired resident, announce each food, allow for sips of liquids, and pace the feeding to conserve energy, ensure safety, and enhance social interaction and satisfaction with meal time.

EXAM ALERT

When assisting to walk, stand beside and slightly behind the resident who is wearing the gait belt snugly around the waist; hold the gait belt with your hands to increase your control and help increase the resident's sense of security.

▶ Always announce when you are leaving the resident's room and make the call light readily available.

▶ Keep eyeglasses, magnifying glass, or other reading devices clean, in good repair, and readily available for the resident; report any damage or loss to the nurse immediately.

▶ If assisting the resident to care for an artificial eye (also called a *prosthesis*), follow the facility's procedure for removing, cleaning, and reinserting it.

Hearing Impairments

Residents with hearing disorders have trouble understanding speech, especially fast speech; they are also confused by noises, echoes, and hollow sounds. They have trouble understanding accented speech by persons for whom English is a second language because they often pronounce syllables and words differently. Although research indicates hearing loss does not directly affect the activities of daily living (ADLs) of hearing-impaired residents, they do report a loss of interest in socializing, which affects their quality of life.

Communication principles to remember when working with hearing-impaired residents include:

▶ Placing yourself directly in front of the resident prior to beginning a conversation

▶ Decreasing as much background noise as possible

▶ Talking in a low tone and in an unhurried manner

EXAM ALERT

High-pitched sounds are especially hard to understand for those with hearing impairments.

- Speaking clearly and distinctly

- Keeping objects out of your mouth when you speak and not covering your mouth when talking

- Making short statements but long enough to help give the resident a frame of reference; for example, "The chaplain *from the First Street Church* is coming for a visit today."

- Using sign language, finger spelling, teaching posters, note pads, white boards, or other visual aids to improve communication

- Restricting conversation to one topic at a time, changing topics carefully, and giving the resident enough time to follow the change

- For the resident who wears a hearing aid device, using the same communication techniques as with other hearing-impaired residents

- Taking special care of hearing aids or other devices and following the facility's procedure for cleaning and storage to prevent damage or accidental losses

- Asking the resident to confirm his or her understanding of important information by repeating instructions

Residents with visual or hearing impairments might have other stronger senses to help offset their loss. For example, touch and smell might be stronger; for the visually impaired resident, the ability to hear might be more acute; for the hearing-impaired resident, sight might help compensate for the hearing loss. In all cases, you should encourage residents to use all the senses, called *sensory stimulation*, or the ability to use one's senses. Likewise, excessive noise, sights, smells, and sounds can overly stimulate some residents. This is known as *sensory overload* and should be avoided, especially when the resident is suffering from undue physical or emotional stress or illness.

Speech Impairment

Remember some general principles for residents who might be dysphasic (have difficulty speaking). This condition can be due to a nervous system disorder such as a stroke (also called a cerebral vascular accident [*CVA*]), Parkinson's disease, Alzheimer's disease, or an injury that affects the speech center in the brain. Other causes of dysphasia might be a result of surgery to remove cancer from the mouth, oral cavity, tongue, or larynx (voice box) affecting speech. These residents might make sounds but cannot form words. Remember that they understand what you are saying because their speech problem has no effect on their intelligence. They often become frustrated by trying to speak clearly and require your patience as you listen to them. Do not hurry them or try to finish what you believe they are trying to say to you. Using assistive devices such as a white board, visual aids, and so on can help ease the frustration of the dysphasic resident who tries hard to communicate. Praise their efforts and encourage them to use every sense they can to convey their needs and actively participate in their daily activities.

> **NOTE**
>
> Always address each resident experiencing vision, hearing, or speech problems with respect. Avoid offensive or demeaning descriptions, such as blind, deaf, mute, or disabled. Instead, use terms such as vision impaired, hearing impaired, or disability.

Respiratory Problems

Residents might experience breathing problems that are short term, or *acute*, such as accidental choking, respiratory arrest, or shortness of breath (also called *dyspnea*) caused by an allergic reaction to a food or drug or by other medical conditions or illnesses. If left untreated, these acute conditions can become terminal. Respiratory complications can lead to *hypoxia*, or a lack of adequate supply of oxygen to the body tissues that damage the brain and the kidneys before other organs. Residents in respiratory distress will struggle to breathe and show signs of *shock*, which causes their skin to turn bluish in color (*cyanosis*), their blood pressure to fall (*hypotension*), and their pulse to rise (*tachycardia*). They will also become confused or combative as they lose oxygen to their brain. If this condition is not corrected, they will stop breathing, a condition called *respiratory arrest*. Respiratory arrest can occur very quickly if residents develop a life-threatening allergic reaction to a food, drug, or insect sting. If you see that the resident is not breathing, call for help and begin *rescue breathing* by delivering two long breaths by mouth to mouth or mask to mouth technique. Continue breathing for the resident at the rate of at least 12 breaths per minute until the resident resumes breathing or until you are relieved. For severe allergic reactions, the nurse will administer emergency drugs. Oxygen is a drug and, as such, must be administered by a licensed nurse. You can support the resident receiving oxygen by observing the resident's response to oxygen therapy; that is, the rate, depth, and ease of his or her respirations, skin color, and alertness.

Residents may receive oxygen therapy for chronic diseases affecting the respiratory system, such as chronic obstructive lung disease (*COPD*), emphysema, or chronic bronchitis. These conditions cannot be reversed and result in a constant struggle to move air in or out of the lungs. Difficult bouts of productive coughing also occur, leaving the resident exhausted. *PCP*, a special type of pneumonia as a complication of Acquired Immunodeficiency Syndrome (AIDS), can be lethal. Other types of pneumonia can also become life threatening to residents already weakened by a chronic illness or condition that affects their ability to heal (referred to as *debilitating*). Surgery also poses a great risk for pneumonia in these residents.

EXAM ALERT

Maintain a safe environment for residents who receive oxygen. Remember to post "Oxygen in Use" signs in the resident's room, warn visitors not to smoke (oxygen supports combustion), and report any change in the resident's condition.

Other considerations in caring for the resident receiving oxygen include the following:

▶ Position the resident to make breathing as effortless as possible.

▶ If confined to bed, change the resident's position every two hours.

▶ Provide mouth care to keep the resident's mouth clean and moist.

▶ Encourage frequent rest periods and arrange activities and care to promote rest.

▶ Follow standard precautions for disposing of sputum.

▶ Observe special precautions for active respiratory infections, including TB.

▶ Observe and record any changes in sputum (changes could indicate infection or bleeding from the lungs).

▶ Observe all safety precautions for the resident receiving oxygen.

▶ Encourage fluids to help thin secretions; clear liquids are best for this purpose.

▶ Encourage proper food intake to maintain nutrition and energy needs.

▶ Provide careful skin care for residents receiving oxygen by any delivery method that uses tubing or with any appliance or equipment with edges that put pressure on the nose (*nares*), the top of the nose, cheeks, or ears.

▶ Keep face masks clean and placed snugly to ensure oxygen delivery.

NOTE

Review the care of the resident receiving oxygen in Chapter 6.

▶ Maintain water in wall oxygen reservoir to keep delivered air moist. Change water according to facility protocol.

▶ If receiving oxygen via portable tank, do not drop or damage the tank, and report any leakage to the nurse; replace the tank to maintain constant oxygen supply.

▶ Provide emotional care to ease the resident's fears of not being able to breathe normally.

▶ Keep the call light within easy reach of the resident.

▶ Observe and report any changes in the resident's breathing pattern.

▶ *Never* adjust or discontinue the oxygen.

Chronic or long-term respiratory problems such as emphysema and chronic bronchitis might lead to *apnea*, or respiratory arrest, which means that the resident stops breathing. The resident will require assistance to breathe artificially with the help of a *mechanical ventilator*. The ventilator enables oxygen and carbon dioxide to be exchanged. The ventilator tubing connects to a *tracheostomy*, or permanent surgical opening into the *trachea*, the air passage from the throat to the lungs. Ventilator-dependent residents must rely on others for their care. Conscious residents might be very frightened by the ventilator and their inability to talk; some might be comatose, or unaware of their surroundings. Special considerations in caring for the ventilator resident are as follows:

▶ Remember that you are caring for a human being, not a machine.

▶ To protect the resident's airway, work with another caregiver to move the resident.

▶ Measure, record, and report vital signs, noting any change in respiratory effort.

▶ Provide personal care and ADLs that protect the resident's airway.

▶ Provide frequent oral care.

▶ Keep the ventilator connected to the electrical outlet, and tubes connected and free of kinks.

▶ Provide for frequent position changes and rest periods to conserve the resident's energy.

▶ Keep the call light within easy reach of the resident and answer it promptly to help allay resident fears.

▶ Speak to the unconscious, comatose resident on a ventilator as though the resident can hear you.

NOTE

Research shows that comatose persons can often hear but cannot communicate.

▶ Offer emotional support.

▶ Immediately report any signs of respiratory difficulty or ventilator alarms to the nurse.

▶ *Never* adjust the ventilator settings or remove a resident from a ventilator.

Cardiovascular Problems

Cardiovascular problems involve the heart and blood vessels.

Heart Disease

Heart disease kills more elders worldwide than any other disease. Diseased blood vessels can prevent adequate blood circulation, which can result in pain, disability, and death. The arteries supplying the heart muscle (*coronary arteries*) can become narrowed (*arteriosclerotic*) over time or blocked by a buildup of *plaque* (a patch inside the artery's lining caused by accumulated fats or calcium, also called *atherosclerosis*). The narrow or blocked artery cannot deliver oxygen to the heart muscle, causing chest pain (*angina*), which can worsen with any type of strenuous activity. Arteriosclerosis is also responsible for a temporary condition in which the resident experiences dizziness, light-headedness, or confusion due to an inadequate supply of oxygen to the brain, known as a transient ischemic attack (*TIA*). The resident is at high risk for falling during a TIA. Should this occur when assisting the resident to walk, stop the walk, ease the resident to the floor, stay with him or her, and call for help. Any condition that causes the blood flow into and outside the heart can also threaten the resident's life. This is one reason why an accurate and thorough description, recording, and reporting of any abnormal pulse rate or rhythm is so important.

> **EXAM ALERT**
>
> A blood clot can develop in a sclerotic coronary artery, stopping the oxygen supply to the heart muscle, which leads to a heart attack, or acute myocardial infarction (AMI). This is a life-threatening emergency requiring emergency care and transportation to the hospital emergency room.

Following a heart attack, the heart is often weakened and loses its ability to pump adequately, which can lead to *congestive heart failure (CHF)*. CHF causes a buildup of fluid in the lungs, resulting in dyspnea and a wet cough or swelling of the extremities (*edema*). A sudden, severe episode of dyspnea, edema, and urine retention can result in death.

Circulatory Conditions

Arteries or veins in the circulation of the lower extremities can also be blocked by a clot (*thrombus*), which can cause swelling, pain, and disability. Signs of *thrombosis* (a blood clot in the vein) include a reddened, warm area in the lower leg, swelling, and pain, which increases with movement.

If a thrombus becomes dislodged from a vein in the lower extremity, it becomes a traveling clot, meaning it moves to the heart, lungs, or brain, causing a heart attack, respiratory distress, or a stroke. Report all resident complaints of sudden pain or dyspnea immediately because these are considered emergencies.

> **CAUTION**
>
> If the resident complains of pain in the lower leg or dyspnea, do not massage the affected leg, ambulate the resident, or bend the toes of the affected leg upward because these movements help to dislodge a clot.

Clots in the arteries of the lower extremity can slow or stop circulation. The resident will complain of pain, coolness, and a pale color in the affected leg, which is a condition requiring immediate surgery to restore adequate circulation.

Hypertension

Hypertension, or high blood pressure, is defined as unusually high blood pressure for an individual, usually exceeding 140/90 after two consecutive readings in the same arm. Hypertensive individuals are more prone to develop heart disease or other medical conditions. Although the cause of hypertension is unknown, diet, obesity, the effects of diabetes, and other lifestyle factors affect blood pressure. Hypertension can affect all body systems, damage organs, and become lethal because it can lead to a stroke. Specialized care of residents with cardiovascular problems or hypertension is similar and includes the following:

▶ Follow the plan of care very carefully to promote healing and prevent further complications.

▶ Provide foods and fluids, and monitor I & O as prescribed to provide energy and prevent edema.

▶ Assist in monitoring the resident's prescribed dietary restrictions regarding salt, fat, sugar, and fluid.

▶ Modify ADLs and care activities to save energy and promote rest.

▶ Provide exercise as tolerated to maintain function and activity level.

▶ Monitor vital signs and report any changes immediately to the nurse.

▶ Provide comfort measures and emotional support.

▶ Closely observe and promptly report any changes in the resident's condition.

Paralysis

Residents might be unable to move a body part, which is called *paralysis*. Paralysis is classified according to how much of the body is affected. For example, paraplegia affects the lower half of the body; *quadriplegia* involves both arms and legs; *hemiplegia* means that half of the body, either the right or the left side, is paralyzed. A stroke or other neurological disease results in decreased blood flow and oxygen to the brain cells, causing them to die, which leads to paralysis. Signs and symptoms of a stroke depend on the location of the brain injury and the amount of the damage. A stroke on one side of the brain affects the opposite side of the body. Effects of a stroke include *aphasia* (being unable to speak), a partial paralysis or weakness of the face (causing drooping of the mouth, eyelid, and so on), or complete paralysis of the arm or leg on the affected side (leaving the arm or leg limp, or *flaccid*). An injury to the spinal cord can cause paralysis of the body below the injury site, leading to paraplegia or quadriplegia. Paralysis in any part of the body can pose problems with mobility and ADLs. Special care is required to keep the affected muscles and tendons functioning as much as possible. Mobility-impaired residents run the risk of *contractures*, or a shortening of the muscles due to lack of exercise or movement, pressure ulcers, and other hazards of immobility; respiratory difficulties, especially pneumonia; and muscle spasms, incontinence (bowel and bladder), and swallowing difficulties (*dysphagia*). Provide special care to residents affected with an injury that caused paralysis to protect them from further complications, and maintain or restore normal functioning by including the following:

▶ Follow each resident's care plan to help residents regain independence.

▶ Maintain a calm, reassuring environment.

▶ Arrange ADLs to promote rest and sleep.

▶ Encourage independence and self-care to promote autonomy.

▶ Show patience and empathy.

▶ Use touch to help orient the resident and show genuine care and concern.

EXAM ALERT

Feed the resident on the unaffected side of the mouth.

▶ Allow the resident with dysphagia plenty of time to chew and swallow.

▶ Be sure that the dysphagic resident swallows food each time it is offered and before continuing with the feeding.

▶ Use thickener with fluids as ordered when feeding the dysphagic resident.

EXAM ALERT

Keep the dysphagic resident upright for at least 30 minutes after feeding.

▶ Perform passive range of motion to all affected extremities.

▶ Assist the resident in bowel and bladder retraining.

▶ Dress and undress the resident's affected side first.

EXAM ALERT

If assisting the stroke patient with hemiplegia to walk with a cane, use the cane on the affected side. When transferring the paraplegic from bed to wheelchair, lock the wheels on the bed and the wheelchair. Keep the bed of the paralyzed resident in its lowest position with wheels locked.

▶ Report any change in the resident's condition.

▶ In all situations requiring your assistance to move a resident, use proper body mechanics: Keep the spine straight, bend your knees, lift with your legs (not your back), and seek assistance as necessary to protect you and the resident.

▶ Use a mechanical lift, as ordered, to assist in lifting residents.

Digestive and Elimination Problems

Diseases or conditions involving the digestive and urinary system can cause *malnutrition* (inadequate intake and use of foods), elimination difficulties, and complications due to infections, cancer, or organ failure.

Infections

Severe infections of the digestive organs include gall bladder disease (*cholecystitis*), *pancreatitis* (inflammation or infection of the pancreas), *hepatitis* (liver infection), or *nephritis*, (kidney disease). Common symptoms include severe pain, nausea, vomiting, fever, diarrhea or constipation, dysuria, or a yellowish color to the skin (*jaundice*), and life-threatening chemical imbalances. Residents may also become confused, which can be mistaken for a psychological event when, in fact, they may be exhibiting the first sign of a urinary tract infection (UTI). Residents recovering from infections might be kept *NPO*, meaning they can have no foods or fluids by mouth. The resident will receive fluids, nutrients, antibiotics, and other medications through an *IV* (within the vein), or intravenous access device. IV therapy provides direct access to the bloodstream through an IV catheter and tubing attached to a sterile bag of fluids; the solution is connected to a pump that controls the amount of fluid delivered. A sterile dressing covers the IV catheter insertion site and must be maintained according to facility procedure. The tasks of starting, adjusting, and discontinuing IV therapy are reserved for the licensed nurse. You can support the resident receiving IV therapy by being careful to not pull on the IV catheter, kink the IV tubing, or interrupt the IV flow.

CAUTION

Do not place the solution below the IV site.

Change the resident's gown or clothing carefully to maintain the IV connection. Immediately report to the nurse any signs of infection, swelling at the IV site, or activation of IV pump alarms.

Cancers in the Digestive and Urinary Tract

Cancerous growths, or *tumors*, can interfere with normal food intake, nutrient use, and elimination of digestive wastes, putting pressure on or within the digestive organs that interferes with normal digestion and circulation. As cancer cells grow, they rob normal cells of nutrients and interfere with normal cell activity. Cancer cells can travel through the body from an original invasion site to a distant organ (*metastasis*), resulting in further damage and, eventually, death. Common sites for metastasis are the brain, bone, and liver.

Residents recovering from surgery to remove a cancerous tumor in the GI tract, bladder, or kidney who cannot swallow or take foods or fluids by mouth (*PO*) might require tube feedings or *total parenteral nutrition (TPN)*. A small tube inserted into the stomach through the nose (*nasogastric tube* or feeding tube) provides short-term nutrition during the healing process. If needed for an extended period, a *gastrostomy tube (G tube)* is inserted directly into the stomach through a *stoma* (a surgical opening in the abdomen). A pump attached to the feeding tube delivers the prescribed amount of food and fluid over time. For safety considerations, an alarm will sound to signal a pump problem. Residents receiving their total diet through a feeding tube are often NPO, or can have no food or fluids by mouth. Be careful to observe this order. It is also important to protect the skin and mucous membranes around the nose or the stoma because they can become irritated. Provide oral care at least every two hours or more, raise the head of the bed at least 35 degrees, and keep the call light in easy reach. Remember to keep the skin around the G tube clean and report any sign of skin breakdown or abdominal discomfort.

Residents recovering from surgery to remove cancer from the bladder, small intestine, or colon (large intestine that holds solid wastes) might also have a temporary or permanent *ostomy*, or surgical diversion to aid in elimination. Diversion means that, in the case of bladder cancer, an artificial appliance is attached to a stoma in the abdomen to provide an alternative path to expel urine. If a portion of the large intestine is removed, an appliance is attached to an abdominal stoma to collect feces/stool (*colostomy*). The resident will need ostomy care training and emotional support to adjust to dramatic changes in urine and bowel elimination that affect body image, especially if the ostomy is permanent.

Chronic Diseases

Chronic liver disease such as *cirrhosis* (scarring of the liver) causes a buildup of toxic wastes in the body due to failure of the liver to handle the chemicals released by metabolism. The liver might eventually fail, which causes lethal consequences in other body systems, including *hemorrhage* from ruptured veins in the esophagus. Treatment for digestive disorders might include dietary restrictions, medications, chemotherapy, or surgery.

Chronic kidney disease, often linked to type I diabetes, affects all body systems and can result in kidney failure. The resident with kidney failure is at increased risk of life-threatening complications, such as congestive heart failure and severe generalized infection, because the kidneys are not able to filter toxins from the body or control fluid and electrolyte absorption. Specialized care of residents with chronic diseases or those recovering from surgery includes the following:

▶ Observing, recording, and reporting vital signs, and pain tolerance

▶ Observing, recording, and reporting any changes in the surgical site

▶ Strictly adhering to the diet order, including fluid restrictions

▶ Keeping feeding tubes free of kinks

▶ Prompt reporting of vomiting, diarrhea, constipation, or skin color changes

▶ Observing, recording, and reporting of *emesis* (vomit) or abnormal stools or urine, especially color, consistency, or odor

▶ Using standard precautions when handling bodily fluids

▶ Prompt emptying and care of stoma appliances

▶ Observing, recording, and reporting I & O

▶ Observing and reporting any behavior changes

CAUTION

Provide careful skin care, especially around stomas.

▶ Providing frequent oral care

▶ Providing comfort measures to help relieve pain and promote rest (position changes, diversion activities, quiet environment, and so on)

▶ Removing noxious odors

▶ Providing emotional support

Diabetes

Diabetes mellitus, a disease of the endocrine system, is listed separately because it affects metabolism, impacts every system of the body, and is becoming an epidemic among Americans. Diabetes mellitus is a disease of the pancreas in which the body cannot use *carbohydrates* (sugars and starches) efficiently. The pancreas cannot produce enough insulin or does not use insulin properly to change carbohydrates to energy. When this occurs, the body burns fats for energy instead, leading to a dangerous imbalance in *ketones*, the product of fat breakdown.

The exact cause of diabetes is unknown, but several factors such as age, obesity, and family history can contribute to developing diabetes. Residents with type 1 diabetes must take insulin to live; those with type 2 diabetes can control their disease with diet and medication. Both types of diabetes require a careful diet that contains the right amount of proteins, fats, and carbohydrates to maintain adequate nutrition and systems functioning. Signs and symptoms of diabetes include excessive thirst, excessive hunger, excessive urination (*polyuria*), weight loss, night sweats, and irritability.

Despite treatment, diabetes can cause blindness, cardiovascular disease, kidney failure, leg ulcers, and nerve damage. Poor circulation due to diabetes can lead to amputation of the leg. Death can result from a diabetic coma, caused by extreme blood sugar (*glucose*) levels such as *hyperglycemia* (abnormally high amounts of glucose in the blood) or by dangerously low blood sugar, called *hypoglycemia*.

EXAM ALERT

It is important to review signs and symptoms of extreme blood sugar levels as outlined in Table 5.1.

You must observe the diabetic resident closely and report any signs of hyperglycemia or hypoglycemia to the nurse immediately so that steps can be taken to reverse these complications.

TABLE 5.1   Blood Sugar Level Signs and Symptoms

Sign or Symptom	Hyperglycemia (High Blood Sugar)	Hypoglycemia (Low Blood Sugar)
Mood	Sluggish and/or confused	Irritable and/or confused
Respirations	Deep; fruity (sweet) breath odor	Shallow
Pulse	Slow or normal	Rapid and weak
Speech	Slurred	No change
Skin	Hot, dry, and flushed	Cold, clammy, and pale

Strict adherence to the diabetic diet is essential to meet caloric needs and control blood glucose levels.

NOTE

Snacks are part of the diet because they are important to maintain a steady supply of glucose to prevent hypoglycemia.

Diabetic residents might have trouble following a restricted diet, eating foods not prescribed, or overeating. Family members or others might supply snacks or forbidden foods, making compliance a challenge for the nursing staff. You must praise and support the efforts of the diabetic resident as well as educating and supporting family members to follow the care plan to promote health and prevent complications. Careful monitoring of food consumption is important to keep the resident safe. Tell the nurse if the resident does not finish the food served during a meal or refuses snacks.

Special care of the diabetic resident includes

► Inspecting the resident's skin daily, paying attention to the feet for decreased sensation or pain (indicates neuropathy, or nerve damage), redness, or a skin break (sign of tissue damage due to poor circulation).

► Inspecting the resident's shoes for items that may be in them before putting them on the resident's feet.

► Keeping the skin and feet clean, dry, and moist; do not apply moisturizing lotion between the toes.

EXAM ALERT

Follow facility policies regarding nail trim for diabetic residents. If allowed, carefully trim toenails to avoid accidental cuts; never remove corns or calluses.

► Avoiding pressure on the feet or toes by tight shoes, socks, or bed linens.

► Serving meals and snacks on time.

► Encouraging the resident to follow the care plan.

► Observing and reporting any changes in condition immediately.

► Protecting the resident from thermal injury due to extreme water temperature. (Diabetic clients often have reduced sensation to temperature caused by nerve damage in the extremities, known as *diabetic neuropathy.*)

► Including the resident in all aspects of care to promote independence, self-esteem, and compliance with the care plan.

► If allowed by state law for your level of practice, monitoring blood sugars as ordered; promptly reporting excessively high or low blood sugar levels to the nurse.

► Assisting the resident to manage stressful situations because increased stress causes a rise in blood sugar levels.

HIV (Human Immunodeficiency Virus) and AIDS (Acquired Immunodeficiency Syndrome)

Residents with *HIV* have been attacked by a virus that robs them of the ability to fight infections. This viral invasion makes them targets for serious illnesses or cancer. Once infected, the HIV is always present. HIV can be transmitted by infected persons who share IV drug needles or have sexual contact. Although transmission of the virus is *not* spread by casual contact (for example, touching, caressing, sneezing or coughing, and so on), caregivers need to use standard precautions to protect themselves when handling the blood or body fluids of the HIV-infected resident, most particularly, to avoid a needle stick or sharps injury. HIV is transmitted by means other than IV drug needles and sexual contact; contact with blood or other body fluids from an infected person, unclean surgical instruments, and transmission from mother to baby in utero and/or breast milk are other modes of transmission. Residents with HIV might develop *AIDS*, a progressive weakening in the HIV resident, which can occur many years after contracting the virus.

AIDS exposes the resident to *opportunistic diseases*, illnesses that take advantage of the resident's weakened immune system. Although there is no cure for HIV/AIDS, residents receive treatment to combat infections, relieve respiratory distress, weakness, and fatigue, decrease pain and discomfort, and promote nutrition. Although medications and treatments are prolonging the life of AIDS residents, the drugs given to treat AIDS have serious side effects, such as nausea, vomiting, and diarrhea.

Residents with AIDS must be protected from infections and exposure to others who might be ill. They should be provided long periods of rest and planned ADLs to preserve energy.

Staff must also follow agency protocol for handling blood and/or body fluids of residents with AIDS. Staff must be very careful with handling sharps to avoid exposure to the resident's blood. If handling sharps, be careful to *never* recap or place used sharps in the trash container. *Always* place used sharps in the sharps container.

The ravaging effects of drug treatment can discourage residents; they need emotional support to help them comply with the medical care plan. Counseling services can help these residents deal with the lack of information about the disease, accept the realities of AIDS, and restore hope. Listening to the resident and being empathetic, caring, and nonjudgmental are essential approaches you must take when caring for these residents. Support of family members, friends, or support groups can also help improve the quality of life for the AIDS resident.

Psychological Problems

Psychological problems, meaning those conditions affecting thought, mood, and behavior, can be as threatening to the health and well-being of residents as physical illnesses. This section reviews those conditions placing the resident at highest risk for psychological distress and, sometimes, physical danger.

Confusion

Residents might become confused for physical or psychological reasons. Any disease or condition that causes hypoxia can lead to confusion. Drug interactions and side effects, hearing difficulty, and reasoning problems might also contribute to confusion. Other causes can include stress and grief, changing routines or living arrangements, hospitalization, and language or cultural factors. Confused residents often tell the same story repeatedly; they live in the past because it is a more familiar time for them and continually repeat the same task such as buttoning their clothes and pacing. They might become frightened and resist care and involvement in activities.

Confused residents might become suspicious of facility staff, accusing them of stealing from them or trying to hurt them or to keep them from leaving the facility. Residents might also experience Sundowner's Syndrome, which means increased confusion or disorientation in the afternoon or evening hours. Confused residents who are ambulatory might wander from the facility and injure themselves or become lost. If confined to the bed or wheelchair, they might try to get up and risk falling or injuring themselves.

It is important to remind the confused resident of who they are, where they are, and the current date and time. This is part of *reality orientation*. Keeping calendars, clocks, and bulletin boards current can support reality for the resident. Sharing current events with the resident can also help. Being acutely aware of environmental hazards that might harm the confused resident and taking every precaution to protect the resident is a priority.

Aggressive Residents

Confused residents who become defensive, aggressive, or combative need your calm demeanor and understanding so that you can find out what is causing the resident's behavior. It is important that you alert the nurse immediately because reporting the incident might help avoid further escalation by the resident and avoid potential harm.

To diffuse the aggressive behavior, leave the situation if you can and return later. Do not argue with the resident or return his or her aggression. Sit down or, if you must stand, turn your body slightly away from the resident with your arms at your side and your hands open; maintain eye contact with the resident. This open stance also enables you to quickly move out of reach of the resident. Keep your voice calm, supportive, and nonthreatening. Using clear, simple language, attempt to "talk them down." Listen carefully, letting the resident know that you are paying attention to what he or she is telling you, and acknowledge the resident's feelings.

Allow the resident to make as many choices as possible to resolve issues, to "save face," and provide the resident with an opportunity to regain self-control. Watch for signs of increased aggression, such as jaw or fist clenching, pacing, crying, or yelling. If the resident becomes violent toward you or others, protect the resident as well as yourself from harm. Special training is often needed to safely restrain the combative resident. Review the facility procedure for restraints as well as the procedure review in Chapter 6. *Never* hit, push, pull, or otherwise retaliate against a resident, despite the provocation; this is considered assault.

Dementias

Dementia is an irreversible, progressive loss of mental function as evidenced by the loss of memory, ability to make judgments, ability to comprehend/understand and learn, ability to carry out tasks or to use language. Residents with dementia lose their ability to socialize, maintain an occupation, or think abstractly or rationally. They become disoriented, meaning they are confused as to who they are, or cannot recall the current date or time. In later stages of the disorder, residents with dementia become agitated, depressed, and suspicious of others (paranoid). They are frightened and frustrated because they try to adjust to their changing world. Dementia is not a part of aging but, when it occurs, it can be devastating to the resident and family, especially when the resident appears healthy but cannot function normally. In the advanced stage, residents become totally incapacitated and can die from complications of immobility.

Dementia can take many forms, but the most common is that associated with Alzheimer's disease, an increasing occurrence with the population served by long-term care. Alzheimer's disease is the most common type of irreversible dementia in persons over age 65, affecting men and women alike. Alzheimer's disease progresses in stages, eventually destroying all mental and physical abilities. In the Alzheimer's resident, confusion results from the resident's decreased cognitive ability, contributing to a lowered ability to manage stress; the resident becomes easily agitated or frustrated and might experience depression when the resident realizes his or her condition is getting worse.

Persons with Alzheimer's disease experience learning difficulties, cannot complete complex tasks, and have trouble concentrating. They get very upset, cry, or become combative with any change in their normal routine or overstimulating events. As the disease progresses, symptoms worsen and losses become more severe, making ADLs, speaking, and activity more difficult. Residents might see or hear things that are not present (hallucinations), think irrationally (delusions), or become suspicious (paranoid). They might wander and lose interest in eating. Anorexia, or loss of appetite, can lead to nutritional deficiencies. Wandering and getting lost can put them in grave physical danger because they are not afraid of road traffic or other environmental hazards. During the late stages of the disease, Alzheimer's residents no longer recognize others and cannot communicate.

NOTE

Family members need support to deal with this loss of recognition by their loved one, which causes them severe psychological pain, sometimes referred to as "the long goodbye."

Eventually, Alzheimer's residents lose their swallowing reflex, become incontinent, lapse into a coma, and die.

Special care of residents with dementia includes

- ▶ Protecting the resident from accidents and injuries

- ▶ Providing a reassuring environment (controlling noise, loud television, radios, and conversation)

- ▶ Keeping the environment clean and uncluttered

- ▶ Using side rails and other assistive devices per facility protocol to protect resident from wandering

- ▶ Maintaining routines to avoid confusion and overstimulation

- ▶ Allowing the resident time to complete tasks and make simple decisions

- ▶ Avoiding disagreements with the resident

- ▶ Gently touching and reassuring the resident who is suspicious; offering simple explanations

- ▶ Reorienting and using distraction for agitated or wandering residents

- ▶ Arranging evening activities to prevent Sundowner's Syndrome

- ▶ Providing emotional support to family and friends

- ▶ Referring family and friends to the nurse for more information on the resident's progress

Recent advances in pharmaceutical research have made medical treatment of Alzheimer's disease more promising.

The Depressed Resident

Depression is listed here as a mood disorder that interferes with normal activity of the resident and is either short-term or chronic in nature. Symptoms of depression include insomnia or excessive sleeping, extreme sadness, crying, fatigue, poor hygiene and grooming, changes in appetite and weight, withdrawing from social activities, and feelings of worthlessness and hopelessness. Losing loved ones, a spouse, friends, and pets, and dealing with chronic or terminal illness can be very stressful for residents, leaving them to mourn, or grieve for the loss of loved ones, declining health, or a past lifestyle. These feelings and reactions are part of the *grief process*, which occurs in stages necessary for adjusting to a loss. They might enter a stage of *denial*, and then become *angry* and *depressed*. They experience other grief stages that include a physical *bargaining stage*, in which a resident might make a promise to self or to God that, if the situation could change, they would do or feel something different to change their life. In the *acceptance stage*, the grieving resident finds peace in accepting the loss and can move on. Not all residents resolve their grief and might go back and forth between the five grief stages. Those who can find acceptance can regain hope and find joy in their lives.

Residents might also regret their loss of independence, their reliance on others, and changes in their primary role as spouse, homemaker, or wage earner. Their new role of widow or widower might be very difficult to assume as well. Chronic health problems and infirmity can further increase their loss of self-esteem as well as worries about their declining health and the prospect of dying. Further, residents might resent being placed in a long-term care facility, acting out their frustration on others, especially family members responsible for the placement decision. Severe depression can lead to serious illness, disability, and suicide. Watch for statements such as, "I might as well be dead," "I'm not good for anything," or "Everybody would be better off without me."

> **CAUTION**
>
> Although you must keep confidential what the depressed resident shares, report immediately any statement that might signal *suicidal ideation*, or thoughts of committing suicide. Likewise, you cannot promise the resident that you will not tell others because doing so would put the resident at risk for harm.

Special care of the depressed resident includes

- ▶ Encouraging the resident to express feelings
- ▶ Being empathetic
- ▶ Encouraging self-care, decision making, and independence
- ▶ Assisting the resident to meet personal care needs (including grooming, eating, and toileting)
- ▶ Encouraging activity to help improve mood
- ▶ Observing warning signs of potential suicide (talking about killing self, describing method and timeline, and giving away belongings)
- ▶ Observing and removing potential hazards in the environment to protect the resident from harming self (including razors, other sharps, cords, and so on)
- ▶ Being realistic with reassurances; avoiding making statements like "Everything's going to be all right."
- ▶ Avoiding judgmental statements like, "You shouldn't be depressed."
- ▶ Encouraging physical activity and socialization to help improve mood

The Terminally Ill Resident

Coming to grips with one's own mortality is a term describing the need to realize that everyone's life is finite, or has a timeline. A normal developmental task of elders is to leave a legacy they can be proud of and to be prepared to face death with as much dignity as possible. For that purpose, the resident might have an *advance directive* such as a *living will*, power of attorney for health care, or a health-care surrogate, which act as legally binding documents outlining allowances and restrictions for treatment and care should they become *terminally ill* (near death) and unable to make decisions for their own care. In such cases, the resident authorizes another person to carry out his or her expressed wishes. The resident's right to make *end-of-life decisions* is protected by law in the *Patient Self-Determination Act*, which gives patients the right to refuse medical or surgical treatment and the right to prepare legally binding advance directives for such purpose.

End-of-life issues can become controversial, especially if family members or loved ones disagree with the resident's wishes. If the resident does not want to be resuscitated in case of respiratory or cardiac arrest, the doctor will write an order for *do not resuscitate*, or *DNR*. It is important to carry out the order. Current research and development to prolong life are legal/ethical issues debated in the legislature as well as the court system. A controversial practice, *euthanasia* (mercy killing) is legal in Oregon as a means to end suffering and promote dignity of terminally ill persons.

Terminally ill residents might receive *hospice care*, specialized treatment by a team of doctors, nurses, therapists, chaplains, and volunteers who provide pain relief, comfort measures (also called *palliative care*), emotional and psychological support, and grief counseling for families as well as *respite* (relief) care for caregivers. Terminally ill residents have a right to the same level of care and comfort as other residents. They deserve to be informed of their condition and to be included in all aspects of their care as much as possible. Often, nursing staff and family ignore the dying resident, "talking over him or her" as though the resident were not present or excluding him or her from conversation. Terminally ill residents must be treated *holistically* (as a complete human being), meaning they deserve to receive optimal physical, psychological, and spiritual support. Physical needs include personal care, comfort measures, pain relief, food, fluids, and ADLs as tolerated. Keeping the resident comfortable is of utmost importance. Many residents might appear depressed and consider suicide when, in fact, they are experiencing intense pain. Do not ignore their reports of pain, and observe closely for other signs of discomfort, especially for residents whose culture does not allow them to complain.

Providing comfort measures, listening to the dying resident, and spending time with him or her are essential in helping to allay fears, which arise more often from not being able to manage pain rather than fear of dying. Perform personal care to promote rest and prevent discomfort or fatigue. Tailor your care to the needs of the dying resident, offering food or fluids, skin and oral care, and assisting with toileting as much as his or her condition will permit. The dying resident receiving strong pain killers (*analgesics*), especially narcotics, might experience constipation; report bowel changes or abdominal discomfort immediately to prevent further complications. Analgesics can also cause confusion, putting the resident at risk for falls. Monitor the resident carefully for any change in alertness that might indicate confusion.

Because talking about death is uncomfortable, caregivers or family members and friends might avoid talking about it and, due to their own fears, might avoid spending time with the dying resident. It is equally important for you to confront your own thoughts and attitudes about dying in order to be effective when caring for the terminally ill resident. If the resident wants to talk about death, listen carefully and respond openly, honestly, and with compassion.

NOTE

Remember that there are no correct answers to many questions about dying; admitting that you do not have an answer to a question is reassuring in its honesty.

Often, the resident is not looking for answers but needs someone to listen. Along with fear of pain is the resident's common fear of dying alone. Although it might be easier to avoid the resident, staying with him or her to provide emotional support is a form of "being in the moment" and "giving of yourself," the most meaningful care you can provide.

Signs of impending death for terminally ill residents include rapid, irregular and shallow respirations, followed by decreased respirations and periods of apnea (*Cheyne-Stokes respirations*). Other signs of impending death include decreased blood pressure; increased, weak pulse; cyanotic lips, nail beds, hands, and feet; ashen, cold skin; loss of gag reflex; and decreased body functions and awareness, which progresses to unconsciousness or coma. Death occurs when the vital signs are absent. You must report these changes immediately to the nurse, staying with the deceased resident until the nurse arrives. When family members or friends visit the resident, respect their need for privacy but offer your condolences and assistance. Other residents might need support to adjust to the loss. Roommates are especially affected. Be honest and open with them but be careful to maintain confidentiality regarding details of the resident's death.

Assisting the nurse, you will provide *postmortem care*, or care provided for the deceased resident, as soon as possible after the family views the body. The procedure, "Assisting with Post-Mortem Care," is described in Chapter 6.

NOTE

You must show the deceased resident the same respect in death that you showed him/her in life.

Exam Prep Questions

1. How can the nursing assistant best ensure the safety of a resident who is legally blind?

   ○ **A.** Keep the call light within easy reach.

   ○ **B.** Keep an overhead light in front of the resident.

   ○ **C.** Speak loudly when addressing the resident.

   ○ **D.** When assisting residents to walk, stand in front of them and hold their hand to guide them.

2. Which of the following is the best way to communicate with a resident who is completely deaf?

   ○ **A.** Speak loudly and clearly.

   ○ **B.** Smile and turn on the television.

   ○ **C.** Write out all communication.

   ○ **D.** Sit next to the resident and speak into his or her ear.

3. Which of the following is not preventative care for a resident receiving oxygen therapy?

   ○ **A.** Provide oral care more frequently.

   ○ **B.** Provide the resident supervision while smoking.

   ○ **C.** Encourage fluids.

   ○ **D.** Provide careful skin care around nares.

4. A resident complains of sudden chest pain and shortness of breath. What is the nursing assistant's first action?

   ○ **A.** Help the resident to sitting position.

   ○ **B.** Call for another nursing assistant's help.

   ○ **C.** Offer the resident a medication for pain relief.

   ○ **D.** Call the nurse immediately.

5. A resident with diabetes wakes up in the middle of the night asking for a snack. What is the best action of the nursing assistant?

   ○ **A.** Check the resident's diet before bringing the snack.

   ○ **B.** Inform the resident that snacks are not served on the night shift.

   ○ **C.** Let the resident know the kitchen staff is not available.

   ○ **D.** Serve the resident his or her breakfast early.

6. Which of the following is the appropriate response of the nursing assistant when a resident complains of dysuria?

   ○ **A.** Encourage the resident to drink more water.

   ○ **B.** Tell the nurse during the end of shift report.

   ○ **C.** Offer the resident cranberry juice with a meal.

   ○ **D.** Report the complaint to the nurse as soon as possible.

7. A resident who is on continuous gastrostomy tube feedings needs to have the linens changed. Which of the following is a necessary action of the nursing assistant to prevent aspiration of the tube feeding liquid?

   ○ **A.** Keep the tube feeding infusing and place the resident in supine position.

   ○ **B.** Ask the nurse to stop the tube feeding and wait 15 minutes before changing the resident to supine position.

   ○ **C.** Keep the tube feeding infusing and place the resident in prone position.

   ○ **D.** Ask the nurse to stop the tube feeding and wait 5 minutes before changing the resident to prone position.

8. What protective equipment should be worn when disposing of emesis?

   ○ **A.** Gown

   ○ **B.** Mask

   ○ **C.** Gloves

   ○ **D.** Goggles

9. Which of the following is not a sign of hypoglycemia?

   ○ **A.** Shallow respirations

   ○ **B.** Cool skin

   ○ **C.** Irritability

   ○ **D.** Slurred speech

10. Which of the following is a form of paralysis?

   ○ **A.** Hemiplegia

   ○ **B.** Hypertension

   ○ **C.** Aphasia

   ○ **D.** Flaccid

11. What is the best action for the CNA who is taking care of a confused resident whose agitation is increasing?

   ○ **A.** Touch the resident frequently while talking to her.

   ○ **B.** Ask other CNAs to help you in case the resident becomes aggressive.

   ○ **C.** Threaten to put restraints on the resident if his behavior does not change.

   ○ **D.** Report the change to the nurse to prevent potential harm to the resident.

12. The scope of practice for a CNA in an emergency includes all of the following except

   ○ **A.** Apply oxygen.

   ○ **B.** Place the resident in the best position for difficulty breathing.

   ○ **C.** Call for help.

   ○ **D.** Stay in the room and provide assistance as directed by the nurse.

Answer Rationales

1. **A.** A call light is to be easy to locate and reach when needed by the resident to call for help. Keeping an overhead light in front of the resident (B) is incorrect because the light source should be behind the resident to prevent a glare effect. Speaking loudly when addressing the resident (C) is incorrect because other senses such as hearing are heightened. When assisting residents to walk, stand in front of them and hold their hand to guide them (D) is incorrect. The nursing assistant should stand beside or slightly behind the resident and gently guide by the elbow.

2. **C.** When a resident is 100% deaf, the only form of communication is written communication. Speaking loudly and clearly (A) and sitting next to the resident and speaking into his or her ear (D) is effective for someone who is partially deaf or hard of hearing. Smiling and turning on the television (C) is an incorrect form of communication for the hearing and the deaf.

3. **B.** A resident on oxygen should not smoke. Providing oral care more frequently (A), encouraging fluids (C), and providing careful skin care around nares (D) are all part of nursing care for a resident on oxygen.

4. **D.** Chest pain can be caused by the resident having a heart attack. The nurse needs to be notified immediately to increase the resident's chance of recovery and survival. Helping the resident to a sitting position (A) is incorrect because the resident should be placed in a position of comfort and one that enables for ease of breathing. Calling for the assistance of another nursing assistant (B) is incorrect because the nurse needs to be notified immediately. Offering the resident a medication for pain relief (C) is incorrect because it is not part of the nursing assistant's role or responsibility.

5. **A.** Checking the resident's diet to verify what the resident may receive for a snack is part of the procedure when feeding a resident. The nursing assistant washes her hands, checks the identification of the resident, and verifies that the proper diet is delivered. Informing the resident that snacks

are not served on the night shift (B), letting the resident know the kitchen staff is not available (C), and serving the resident his or her breakfast early (D) involve not allowing resident choices, freedom, or involvement in care.

6. **D.** Dysuria is the term used to describe painful urination. Dysuria can be caused by infection or obstruction. Telling the nurse during the end of shift report (B) is incorrect because pain should always be reported as soon as possible. Encouraging the resident to drink more water (A) and offering the resident cranberry juice with a meal (C) are related to the care of a urinary tract infection, but that determination is made by the physician.

7. **B.** The head of the bed is to be at 30–45° while feeding is infusing. When changing position, the nursing assistant is to ask the nurse to turn the tube feeding off and wait 15 minutes before moving the resident. Keeping the tube feeding infusing and placing the resident in supine position (A) and keeping the tube feeding infusing, and placing resident in prone position (C) are incorrect because the tube feeding is still infusing when the position is changed and could lead to aspiration of tube feeding liquid. Asking the nurse to stop the tube feeding and wait 5 minutes before changing the resident to prone position (D) is the incorrect position to change bed linen, and it does not state the correct time of 15 minutes.

8. **C.** Gloves are the only protective equipment needed when emptying an emesis basin. A gown (A), a mask (B), and goggles (D) are not necessary.

9. **D.** Slurred speech is a sign of hyperglycemia. Shallow respirations (A), cool skin (B), and irritability (C) are signs of hypoglycemia.

10. **A.** When a resident suffers a stroke, it could lead to paralysis. The paralysis can involve hemiplegia or quadriplegia. Hypertension (B) is high blood pressure and could lead to a stroke. Aphasia (C) and flaccidity (D) can result from a stroke.

11. **D.** It is important that you alert the nurse immediately because reporting the incident might help avoid further escalation by the resident and avoid potential harm. Actions (A) and (C) may increase agitation. Action (B) is consider false imprisonment, threatening to do harm, and having the ability to carry it out.

12. **A.** The CNA's scope of practice does not include the application of oxygen; it is considered a drug and must be administered by licensed persons only. Answers B, C, and D are within the CNA's scope of practice.

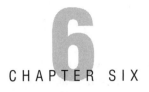

CHAPTER SIX

Clinical Skills Performance Checklist

This chapter reviews the clinical skills most likely to be required in the clinical performance portion of the certification examination, the Clinical Skills Test (CST). Content includes principles of safe practice, the steps needed to perform each skill, and exam alerts you need to recall when answering questions regarding nursing skills on the written examination (WE).

You observe principles of safe practice in providing both indirect and direct care during the CST.

> ▶ **Indirect Care:** Represents performance that is a *part of every skill*; that is, handwashing, ensuring the resident's privacy and comfort, resident rights, safety, and standard precautions (infection control and recording/reporting). You receive a separate score for these skill requirements. The evaluator observes your indirect care performance according to the following checkpoints, or *critical steps*, throughout each skill:
>
> Wash hands before and after each nursing procedure and between direct care given to each resident.
>
> Greet resident, address by name, and introduce self.
>
> Provide explanations to resident before beginning and throughout the procedure.
>
> Provide privacy for the resident: close door or cubicle curtain and protect body from undue exposure.
>
> Promote resident safety: Identify resident; position to protect from falling; use assistive devices as needed; ensure all equipment is in proper working order; lock wheels of bed, wheelchair, stretcher, or other equipment with wheels when transferring resident from one area to another; remain with the resident throughout the procedure to protect from injury; leave call light within easy reach of the resident when leaving the resident's room; provide instructions for post-procedure care as needed to ensure resident safety.

Promote resident rights: right to information regarding purpose of the procedure and findings as needed; dignity as well as observing the resident's right to refuse the procedure.

Use standard precautions; unless otherwise noted, remove your gloves before recording the procedure.

Assemble all supplies at the bedside.

NOTE

If gloves are to be removed and reapplied during the procedure, the action is included in the steps of the skill.

Promote resident comfort: position, adjust room temperature, remove noxious odors as soon as possible, and so on.

Record the procedure, results, and resident's response on the required form.

Report any abnormal results, changes in resident's condition or problems encountered during the procedure to the nurse immediately.

Clean and store equipment, and ensure it is in working order.

Replenish bedside supplies and keep the work area and resident's room tidy.

▶ **Direct Care:** Refers to the particular steps of each separate skill reviewed in the following section. For example, indirect care guidelines related to measuring the radial pulse are the same as for all the skills listed in this chapter. However, the steps for measuring the pulse are different from those involved in measuring the resident's temperature, for example. The evaluator observes and compares the direct care you provide the actor/client to the checkpoints that compose each skill.

Please review the following checklists for the nursing skills you might be required to perform, and practice them until you feel proficient, paying particular attention to the checkpoints and critical steps listed in each skill, because they might be weighted by the evaluator according to how critical each checkpoint is to the safety of the client.

EXAM ALERT

Indirect care checkpoints are included in each skill but are not repeated throughout the documentation of each skill to avoid redundancy. In preparing for the CST, include the indirect skill standards each time you review the skill to reinforce their importance. Checkpoints are likely to be asked on the written examination. Written Exam alerts (the icon that looks like a book) are highlighted here for your review as well.

Handwashing

Checkpoint Critical Step:

1. Wet hands with warm water and apply soap.

2. Work up lather, cleansing front and back of hands, wrists, between fingers, around cuticles, and under nails.

3. Apply friction for a minimum of 30 seconds (as long as it takes to sing "Happy Birthday" twice).

4. Keeping fingers lower than wrist, remove all soap.

5. Dry hands with paper towel and limit contact of towel to cleansed hands; turn off water with fresh, dry paper towel and dispose it of.

6. Complete skill without contaminating hands.

Measuring Body Temperature

Obtain temperature reading per method used as documented in the sections that follow for oral, rectal, axillary, and tympanic modes.

Oral Temperature Measurement with Electronic Monitor

1. Remove thermometer pack from charger and attach oral probe to thermometer.

2. Slide disposable plastic probe cover over thermometer probe until the cover stays in place.

3. Ask resident to open mouth; gently place thermometer probe under side of the tongue to the back of the mouth.

4. Ask resident to close mouth around probe with lips closed.

5. Remove probe when you hear an audible beep and see the temperature display on the thermometer.

6. Push ejection button on thermometer to discard plastic probe cover into appropriate receptacle.

7. Clean equipment as needed after use.

8. Return thermometer probe to recording unit.

9. Return thermometer to the charger.

10. Record temp and mode used to obtain the temp according to agency policy.

Rectal Temperature Measurement with Electronic Thermometer

1. Raise side rail and place resident in Sim's (left side-lying) position.

2. Expose buttocks, keeping rest of body covered.

3. Remove thermometer pack from charger and attach rectal probe to thermometer.

4. Slide disposable plastic probe cover over thermometer probe until the cover stays in place.

5. Dip probe into liberal amount of lubricant applied to a tissue, covering the probe at least 1 to 2 inches.

6. With nondominant hand, separate buttocks to expose anus; ask the resident to breathe slowly and relax.

7. With dominant hand, insert thermometer probe gently into anus, aiming the probe in the direction of the umbilicus, which is 1–2 inches; DO NOT FORCE the probe. If you feel resistance with the probe, withdraw it and notify the nurse.

8. Gently hold thermometer probe in place and remove it when you hear an audible beep and see the temperature display on the thermometer.

9. Push ejection button on thermometer to discard plastic probe cover into appropriate receptacle.

10. Return thermometer probe to recording unit.

11. Wipe the charger and probe with alcohol daily.

12. Return thermometer to the charger.

13. Wipe resident's anal area with tissue to remove lubricant or feces, and discard the tissue in a biohazard receptacle.

14. Record temp and mode used to obtain the temp according to agency policy.

Axillary Temperature with Electronic Thermometer

1. Remove thermometer pack from charger and attach oral probe to thermometer.

2. Slide disposable plastic probe cover over thermometer probe until the cover stays in place.

3. Raise resident's arm away from torso.

4. While holding thermometer horizontal to the resident's axilla, insert thermometer probe into center of axilla, lower arm over probe, and place arm across resident's chest.

5. Remove the thermometer probe when you hear an audible beep and see the temperature display on the thermometer.

6. Push ejection button on thermometer to discard plastic probe cover into appropriate receptacle.

7. Clean equipment as needed.

8. Return thermometer probe to recording unit.

9. Record temp and mode used to obtain the temp according to agency policy.

Tympanic Membrane Temperature with Electronic Thermometer

1. Request the resident to position head to one side away from you.

2. Note if there is cerumen (earwax) visible in the ear canal opening; do not attempt to remove cerumen from inside the outer ear canal.

3. Remove handheld thermometer unit from charger.

4. Apply speculum cover over the tip of the unit (speculum), twisting the cover until it is securely in place.

5. Gently pulling ear pinna (soft lower tip of the ear) up and outward, insert speculum (tip of the thermometer unit) into the ear canal opening until it fits snugly into the canal.

6. Leaving speculum in place, depress the thermometer button to measure the temperature.

7. Leave speculum in place until you hear an audible signal and see the temperature measure on the digital display.

8. Gently remove the speculum.

9. Push ejection button on thermometer to discard plastic speculum cover into appropriate receptacle.

10. Return thermometer to charger.

11. Clean equipment as needed.

12. Record temp and mode used to obtain the temp according to agency policy.

Measuring the Radial and Apical Pulse

Radial Pulse

Checkpoint Critical Step:

1. Place resident in the supine or sitting position.

2. If the resident is lying supine, place arm straight at side or fold arm over chest; if sitting, support arm with your arm or place on flat surface.

3. Place fat pads (just below finger tip) of first two fingers over groove along thumb (radial) side of resident's wrist; slightly extend the wrist.

4. Lightly press against the radial bone until the pulse is absent momentarily, and then release pressure to feel the strongest pulse.

5. Determine the strength of the pulse: pounding-bounding (+4), strong (+3), weak (+2), thready (+1), or absent (0).

6. If the pulse rate is irregular or less than 50 beats per minute (BPM), count the pulse for 60 seconds.

7. Count the pulse for 30 seconds; multiply the total count by 2. If pulse is irregular (less than 50BPM or over 100BPM), notify the nurse.

8. Record results according to agency policy.

EXAM ALERT

A pulse rate less than 50–60 can indicate a serious condition and should be reported to the nurse immediately.

9. Record the rate, strength, and rhythm of the radial pulse on the facility form.

Apical Pulse

1. Clean earpieces and diaphragm of stethoscope.

2. Assist resident to supine or sitting position. Expose sternum (breastbone) and left side of chest.

3. With two or three fingers of your hand, locate the point of maximum intensity (PMI or apical pulse) of the heartbeat on the left chest wall.

4. Place the diaphragm of stethoscope over PMI and auscultate (listen) to the heartbeat for 30 seconds and multiply the count by 2; if the pulse is irregular, listen for 60 seconds.

5. Reposition resident's gown or clothing over chest area and clean ear pieces and diaphragm of stethoscope.

6. Record the rate, strength, and rhythm of the apical pulse on the facility form.

EXAM ALERT

For testing purposes, count the apical pulse for 60 seconds.

Measuring the Respirations

1. Place resident in supine or sitting position; be sure you can view the chest.

2. Place resident's arm across the chest comfortably, keeping your hand on the chest or the upper abdomen.

3. While talking to the resident to provide distraction, observe complete respiratory cycle (one inspiration and one expiration); while watching the sweep hand on your watch, count respirations for 30 seconds; multiply the count by 2.

4. If the respirations are irregular, count them for 60 seconds.

EXAM ALERT

For testing purposes, count respirations for 60 seconds

5. Record respiratory effort (unlabored to labored), depth (shallow to deep), and rate on the facility form.

Blood Pressure

1. Position the resident in supine or sitting position; if the resident has been active, wait at least five minutes before measuring the blood pressure.

2. If resident is sitting, make sure both feet are flat on the floor; no crossed legs.

3. Ask the resident to avoid talking because talking can increase blood pressure by 10–15 mmHg.

4. Select proper size blood pressure cuff (sphygmomanometer). The cuff should fit 40% of the upper arm (if cuff is too small, the reading will be falsely high; if too large, the reading will be a false low reading).

5. Locate brachial artery (in bend of elbow on the side closest to the resident).

6. Place the cuff snugly around the upper arm approximately two-finger widths above the elbow.

7. Position the resident's arm at the level of the heart if sitting or at the resident's side while lying.

8. If a dial is connected to the cuff, place the cuff so the dial is easily seen.

9. Place the bell of the stethoscope diaphragm over the brachial artery and hold snugly with the fingers of your nondominant hand; avoid touching the resident's clothing or blood pressure cuff with the stethoscope.

10. Close valve of the cuff pump clockwise until tight.

11. Quickly inflate the cuff (around 8 seconds) to within 30 mmHg above estimated systolic pressure.

12. Slowly release pressure valve, deflating the cuff, and allow needle of manometer gauge to fall at the rate of 2 to 3 mmHg/second.

13. Listen for the first clear sound and the point on the gauge at which you heard the first sound.

14. If you become distracted and miss the point on the gauge where the first sound was heard, slowly and completely remove the cuff; wait at least one minute and repeat the procedure.

15. Continue to slowly deflate the cuff, noting the point at which the muffled sound completely disappears.

16. Listen as the needle moves 10 to 20 mmHg beyond the last sound and allow the cuff to completely deflate.

NOTE

If measuring the blood pressure for the first time, measure the blood pressure in both arms and record the second set of measurements as the baseline. For subsequent measurements, use the arm with the highest initial reading. Avoid taking the blood pressure in the affected arm of the resident who has had a mastectomy or the arm in which a dialysis shunt or IV is located.

17. Remove cuff and return resident to comfortable position.

18. Record blood pressure according to agency policy.

Partial Bedbath

1. Check to be certain water is at a safe and comfortable temperature.

2. Drape resident so that only the area of the body being bathed is exposed.

3. Use washcloth without soap to cleanse the face.

4. Wipe eyes from inner canthus (side of eye closest to the nose) to the outer canthus (side of eye closest to the ear); change to a clean area of washcloth before cleansing other eye.

5. Pat face dry.

6. Protect bedding by repositioning towel under resident while bath procedure is in progress.

7. Using small amount of soap on washcloth, wash neck, hands, arms, and chest.

8. Dry neck, hands, arms, and chest.

9. Assist resident to turn safely to the side; wash, rinse, and dry back.

10. Warm lotion between your hands; apply lotion to the resident's back.

11. Provide backrub from base of spine up to neck and shoulders using gentle, circular strokes.

12. Replace gown without exposing resident, and secure it.

NOTE

For testing purposes, perform a partial bedbath.

Perineal Care of the Female Resident

1. Prepare a basin with comfortable, safe water temperature and place at the bedside.

2. Using a soapy washcloth, cleanse the genital area (urinary meatus, vulva, and perineum), washing from front to back, beginning over the urinary meatus (opening to allow voiding).

3. Using a different portion of the washcloth for each stroke, wipe each side of the vulva (area around the vaginal opening).

4. Cleanse the perineum (from bottom of vaginal opening to anus) from top to bottom.

5. Using a fresh washcloth for rinsing, completely remove all soap from the genital area.

6. Dry the perineal area from front to back.

7. Replace the water if it becomes cold or soapy.

8. Place the resident on side for cleansing of buttocks and rectal area.

9. Thoroughly rinse and dry buttocks and rectal area.

10. Place dry pad underneath resident when procedure is complete.

11. Clean and store equipment and leave work area tidy.

12. Report your observations, noting any redness, irritation, discharge, or pain in the perineal or buttocks area.

Nail Care (Fingers and Toes)

1. Soak nails in warm water at safe, comfortable temperature for 10–20 minutes before cleaning under the nails.

2. Use orangewood stick or wooden end of a cotton swab to remove debris from under the nails.

3. Dry residents' hands or feet after soaking.

4. Keep nail edges smooth; use emery board to file until smooth.

SAFETY NOTE

CNAs do *not* cut toenails because of the possibility of injury/infection. Notify the nurse if the resident needs toenails to be trimmed.

---

5. Apply lotion to residents' hands or feet after nails are manicured; do not apply lotion between toes.

   After massaging hands with lotion, or applying lotion to feet, blot excess lotion with a dry towel. Dry between toes with towel to remove any lotion that may have collected there.

6. Clean and store equipment and leave work area tidy.

7. Report any breaks in skin to the nurse.

Mouth (Oral) Care

1. Position resident in Fowler's position.

2. Protect clothing from accidental spills.

3. Moisten toothbrush with water and apply toothpaste.

4. Brush all surfaces of teeth, sides of the tongue, and gums with gentle motions.

5. Offer resident the opportunity to rinse mouth or, if unconscious or unable to rinse mouth, apply mouthwash with a swab to gums, tongue, and mucous membranes in the mouth.

6. Dry lips and area around mouth.

7. Report any bleeding or presence of lesions (sores) of the mouth to the nurse.

Mouth (Oral) Care: Care of Dentures

1. Keep dentures in a denture cup or emesis basin for transport to the sink for cleansing.

2. To reduce the risk for denture breakage, fill the sink with water or pad it with a paper towel.

3. Using cool or tepid running water, hold the dentures over the sink and thoroughly clean and rinse them.

4. Store clean dentures in denture cup filled with clean, cool, or tepid water.

5. Using a toothbrush or swab, provide mouth care to resident.

6. Offer resident the opportunity to rinse mouth.

7. Don clean gloves and inspect the inside of the mouth for lesions, redness, or sore areas.

8. Report any redness, irritation, sores, or pain in the resident's mouth.

Dressing

1. Encourage resident to choose clothing to wear.

2. Collect all garments before removing gown or soiled clothing.

3. If one side of body is weak or paralyzed, support affected arm/side while undressing and dressing.

4. Remove gown or soiled garment from affected arm last.

5. Gather sleeve in hands and ease over affected arm.

6. Assist resident to don pants, shirt with sleeves, and socks.

7. Move extremities gently, being careful not to overextend or force extremities when undressing and dressing.

8. Adjust garments for comfort, alignment, and neat appearance.

9. Place soiled garments in hamper.

Applying Elastic Support Hose

1. Apply the support hose to clean legs while resident is lying in bed.

2. Holding the heel of the stocking, gather the rest of the stocking in your hand.

3. Support the resident's foot at the heel.

4. Slip the front of the stocking over the toes, and then the foot before the heel.

5. Pull the stocking up smoothly over the leg.

6. Keep hose straight and wrinkle-free.

7. Remove the hose at least twice daily (once for bathing), and inspect the feet and legs for edema or reddened areas.

8. Report any signs of poor circulation or discomfort to the nurse.

Making an Occupied Bed

1. Check care plan for any precautions needed in moving and positioning the resident.

2. Adjust bed height to comfortable working condition.

3. Lower the side rail on the side where you are working.

4. Loosen the top bed linens at the foot of the bed.

5. Remove the bedspread and blanket separately; if soiled, hold linen away from uniform and place in a linen hamper. Never place linen on the floor.

6. Cover resident with bath blanket: Place blanket over resident and, with the resident holding the blanket in place (if unable to hold, tuck the top edge under the resident's shoulder), bring top sheet down to resident's ankles and remove from the bed; place in hamper.

7. Checking to be certain side rail on opposite side of the bed is up, ask the resident to roll onto side facing away from you (if resident is unable to assist, ask a coworker to roll resident toward opposite side).

8. Loosen bottom sheet and slide sheet from head of the bed, beneath resident, to the foot of the bed on the side nearest you.

9. Replace side rail up on side and move to opposite side of the bed. Repeat step 8.

10. With seam side down (facing the mattress), fanfold the pull sheet toward the back of the resident and tuck just under the shoulders, back, and buttocks; proceed to fanfold the bottom sheet and tuck; follow with the mattress pad, if changing it.

11. Clean, disinfect, and thoroughly dry the exposed mattress surface, if soiled.

12. Apply clean linen to the exposed side of the bed, mattress pad first, placing the center creases lengthwise along the center of the bed and fanfold other half toward the resident; repeat the same maneuver with the bottom sheet, and then the pull sheet; smooth all linen surfaces on your side.

13. Assist the resident to roll toward you and remain positioned on the side facing you, explaining that the resident will feel a bump as he or she rolls over the linens in the bed.

14. Raise the side rail on your side of the bed and move to the opposite side.

15. Loosening linens, reach across bed toward the resident and remove soiled linens by folding them into a bundle with soiled side turned inward; place them in the linen hamper.

16. Clean, disinfect, and thoroughly dry the exposed mattress surface, if soiled.

17. Gently pull clean linens smoothly over edge of mattress from head to foot of the bed, beginning with bottom sheet, and then pull sheet.

18. Tuck edges of pull ends of fitted bottom sheet to fit under the mattress.

19. Grasp edges of pull sheet and, leaning backward with spine straight, pull sheet edges toward you and tuck them snugly under the mattress; smooth all surfaces.

20. Assist resident in returning to supine position.

21. Apply top sheet over bath blanket, placing the length of sheet over client with center crease in the middle of the bed; open the sheet from head to toe and, asking the resident to hold the top hem or tucking it under resident's shoulder, remove bath blanket and place in linen hamper.

22. Tuck bottom edge of top sheet under the mattress; miter the corners.

23. Place blanket or spread over client in same manner as top sheet without the bath blanket in place; keep bottom long edge the same as the edge of the top sheet, usually 6–8 inches from the mattress edge.

24. Turn back top sheet to make cuff over top of the blanket or spread; smooth blanket or spread.

25. Raise the side rails per facility policy.

26. Supporting resident's head, remove pillow and change pillow case; place soiled case in linen hamper; replace pillow to support/align neck and head and for comfort.

27. Place call light within easy reach.

28. Lower the bed position to its lowest level.

29. Remove all soiled linen from the room to designated collection area.

30. Report any reddened areas noted on skin while changing linens.

For all the following positions, move the resident in alignment for safe turning.

Moving the Resident to the Side of the Bed

1. Adjust the bed to a comfortable working height, as flat as possible, and lock the wheels.

2. Raise the side rail on the opposite side prior to lowering the side rail closest to you.

3. Stand with your feet apart (one foot in front of the other), back straight, and knees bent.

4. Cross the resident's arms across the chest.

5. Place your arms under the neck and shoulders; move the area from the shoulders up to the head of the resident's body toward you; shift your weight from one leg to another.

6. Place your arms under the resident's waist and thighs; move the middle portion (torso) of the resident's body toward you.

7. Place your arms under the resident's legs and move the lower portion of the body toward you.

8. If leaving the resident in the changed position, support head and back with pillow.

9. Check the resident for comfort.

10. Lower the bed and raise the side rails, if ordered.

11. Place the call light within easy reach.

Supine Position

1. Position resident on the back with face up, arms at sides, and legs straight and slightly apart.

2. Provide pillows for head and neck support and comfort.

Fowler's Position

1. Raise head of bed at least 30 degrees (low Fowler's position) up to 90 degrees (high Fowler's position).

2. Unless prohibited, raise the knee gatch of the bed to comfort level to keep knees flexed to prevent resident from slipping down in the bed.

3. Support arms as needed for comfort.

Figure 6.1 illustrates the Fowler's position.

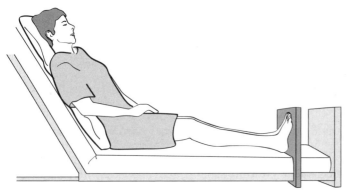

FIGURE 6.1   Fowler's Position

Lateral (Side-Lying) Position

1. Raise the opposite side rail and lock the wheels.

2. Move the resident to the side of the bed nearest you.

3. Flex the resident's distant arm from you next to the head and place the resident's arm nearest you across the chest.

4. Cross the resident's leg nearest you over the other leg at the ankle.

5. Place one hand on the resident's shoulder and the other hand on the nearest hip.

6. Turn the resident away from you onto the side.

7. Use a positioning device; add a pillow folded lengthwise against the resident's back to provide back support.

8. Use a positioning device; add a pillow under uppermost leg from knee to below foot.

9. Adjust resident's arm and shoulder to avoid pressure.

10. Provide positioning device; add a pillow to support shoulder and arm.

11. Lower the bed and the side rail as ordered.

Figure 6.2 illustrates a lateral position.

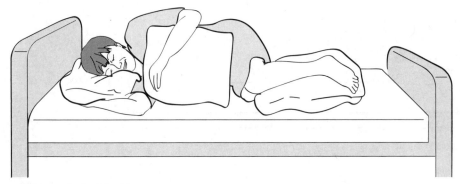

FIGURE 6.2 Lateral Position

Sim's Position

The Sim's position is the same as the lateral position but with the undermost arm positioned at the resident's back. Figure 6.3 illustrates a Sim's position.

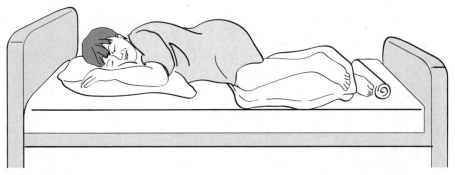

FIGURE 6.3 Sim's Position

Prone Position

1. Position the resident on abdomen with face turned to one side; position arms straight or flexed upward toward the head.

2. Keep the bed as flat as possible.

Figure 6.4 illustrates a prone position.

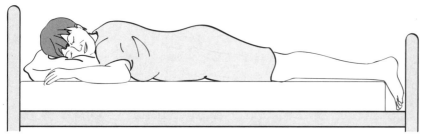

FIGURE 6.4 Prone Position

Orthopneic Position

1. Assist the resident to sit straight up or assume a sitting position on the side of the bed.

2. Place a pillow on the overbed table and move the table directly under the upper body of the resident.

3. Assist the resident to lean forward and place both arms, slightly bent, at the elbows, on the pillow for comfort.

Figure 6.5 illustrates an orthopneic position.

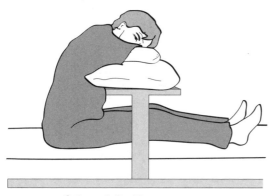

FIGURE 6.5 Orthopneic Position

Logrolling the Resident

1. Using correct body mechanics, raise the side rails; raise the bed to a comfortable working position and lock the wheels.

2. Keeping the bed as flat as possible, lower the side rail on your working side.

3. Roll the pull sheet placed under the resident up close to the resident's body.

4. Place a pillow between the resident's knees.

5. Hold the pull sheet at the resident's shoulders closest to you (the other nursing assistant holds the hip) and move the resident to your working side of the bed.

6. Raise the side rail closest to you; you and your assistant must move to the other side of the bed; stand at the resident's shoulders; your assistant stands near the thighs.

7. Lower the side rail closest to you.

8. Working together, grasp the pull sheet at the resident's shoulders and hips and, as the resident holds himself or herself stiffly, turn the resident in one smooth movement to keep the spine straight.

9. Place the resident in side-lying or Sim's position.

10. Place pillow behind head and neck for resident comfort.

11. Lower the bed and raise the side rails, if ordered.

12. Place the call light within easy reach.

Figure 6.6 illustrates how to logroll a resident.

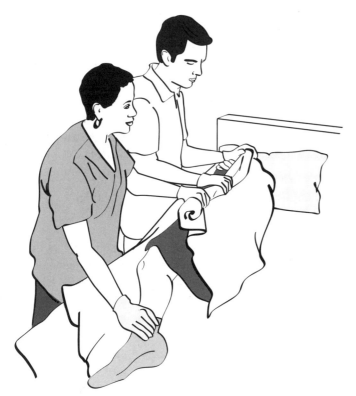

FIGURE 6.6 Logrolling a Resident

Assisting the Resident to Sit on the Side of the Bed

1. Position the bed so that the resident's feet can either touch the floor or a footstool.

2. Raise the side rail behind the resident.

3. Assist the resident to a sitting position.

4. Place one arm behind the resident's neck and shoulders; place the other arm under the resident's knees. Raise the head of the bed to a 90 degree angle.

5. Turn the resident toward you so his or her legs hang over the side of the bed.

6. Support the resident while he or she regains balance.

7. Ask resident if he/she is experiencing dizziness or nausea. Encourage the resident to keep his/her head erect with the eyes open. Note that if the resident wears glasses for distance vision, make sure the resident has them on throughout the procedure.

8. Stay with resident to support an upright position, keeping body in straight alignment.

9. Check pulse and respirations.

10. Allow the resident to remain in the dangling position for 15–20 minutes or as ordered.

11. Return the resident to bed by reversing the process.

Assisting the Resident to Transfer from the Bed to a Chair or Wheelchair

1. Place the chair next to the bed on the resident's strong side.

2. If using a wheelchair, lock the wheels and fold the footrests to the outside of the chair.

3. Place the bed in the lowest position and lock the wheels.

4. If side rails are up, lower the one nearest you.

5. Assist the resident to put on nonskid shoes and a robe.

6. Assist the resident to sit on the side of the bed and dangle to ensure balance. If using a gait-transfer belt, apply it snugly around the waist with belt buckle in front.

7. Place nonskid footwear on resident's feet before standing to prevent sliding of resident's feet on floor.

8. With your arms under the resident's axilla, assist the resident to push down on the mattress and, on the count of three, stand facing you, blocking the resident's knees and feet with yours; if using a gait-transfer belt, grasp the belt from underneath at each side.

9. Taking small steps or turn together (pivot) to a position so that the resident's back of the knees touches the front of the chair.

10. Ask the resident to grasp the arms of the chair or your forearms and, on the count of three, bend your knees and lower the resident into the chair.

11. Place the call light within the resident's reach.

To assist the resident to transfer from a chair or wheelchair to a bed, simply reverse the preceding steps.

Transferring the Resident from a Bed with a Mechanical Lift

Figure 6.7 illustrates some mechanical lifts that you might use to transfer the resident, as documented in the list that follows.

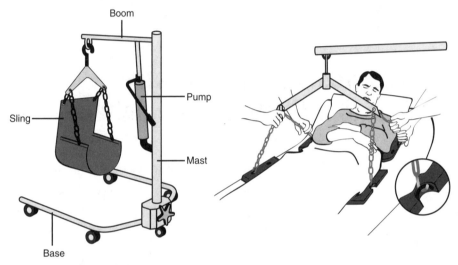

FIGURE 6.7 Mechanical Lifts

1. Ask for assistance to operate the lift.

2. Gather the lift and all supplies at the bedside.

3. Wheel the lift into position with the foot extensions under the bed on the side where the chair is positioned.

4. Set the adjustable base at its widest setting to assure its stability. Lock the wheels of the lift.

5. Secure the lifting chains to handles on the side of the lift sling.

6. Place the lift sling under the resident, placing the narrow end at the top of the shoulders and the wider end to below the knees; center the resident's body on the sling to provide for equal distribution of weight.

7. Move the lift arms directly over the resident and lower the horizontal bar by releasing the hydraulic valve; when the lift arms are in place, close the valve.

8. Attach the lift straps or hooks to the openings on the lift seat and gradually lift the resident above the bed surface.

9. As you continue to operate the lift, ask a coworker to guide the resident with his or her hands as the client is lifted, checking to be sure the sling is securely under the resident.

10. Move the client over the chair making certain that the hydraulic valve is *closed*.

11. Releasing the hydraulic valve very slowly and smoothly, lower the client into the chair.

12. Secure the resident throughout the lift for protection and reassurance.

13. Following the lift into the chair, wheelchair, or stretcher, leave the sling under the resident for easy return to bed as ordered.

14. Apply seat belt or other restraint as needed.

15. Place the call light within easy reach.

16. When the resident returns to bed, follow the same process for operating the lift and, when the resident is positioned in bed, remove the sling.

17. Clean and store the lift per facility policy.

Moving the Resident from a Bed to a Stretcher (Gurney)

1. Ask for assistance from two or three coworkers.

2. Raise the bed to a comfortable working height and lock the wheels.

3. Remove the top linen and cover with a bath blanket; loosen the pull sheet.

4. If the side rail is up, lower it on your side.

5. Grasp the pull sheet at the resident's shoulder's and waist; ask another coworker positioned next to you to grasp the sheet at the hips and thighs. In unison on the count of three, pull the resident toward you to the side of the bed.

6. Position the stretcher against the side of the bed closest to you at the same height as the bed and lock the wheels.

7. With two other coworkers stationed on the other side of the bed, roll the edges of the pull sheet close to each side of the resident.

8. While two other coworkers steady the resident from the other side of the bed, in unison on the count of three, move the resident from the bed to the stretcher.

9. Position the resident in the center of the stretcher, support the head and shoulders with pillows if allowed, and secure the resident with safety straps and raise the side rails on the stretcher.

10. Unlock the wheels on the stretcher and transport the resident feet first with the help of another coworker.

11. Remain with the resident until relieved by another staff member.

Using a Gait-Transfer Belt to Assist the Resident to Ambulate

1. Apply the gait-transfer belt snugly around the resident's waist, fastening the buckle in the front, slightly to the side, and over the clothing as illustrated in Figure 6.8.

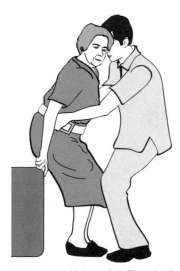

FIGURE 6.8 Using a Gait-Transfer Belt

2. Stand directly in front of the resident with legs slightly apart.

3. While holding the gait-transfer belt with your hands, assist the resident to a standing position so that the resident's feet are positioned between yours.

4. Transfer one of your hands to the side of the gait-transfer belt; move the other hand to hold the belt in the back.

5. Check to be sure the resident has on non-skid footwear, is covered with a robe or clothing, and is wearing distance vision glasses if applicable.

6. To ambulate the resident, keep hands in current position and walk at the resident's side and slightly behind his or her knees.

7. Check frequently to see if resident is feeling unsteady, experiencing dizziness, nausea, or pain.

8. At the completion of the ambulation, return the resident to the chair or bed. If the resident begins to fall, **do not attempt to prevent the fall** but, with your feet wide apart to maintain your balance, bend your knees and lower the resident to the floor. Place your leg behind the resident, allowing the resident to rest his or her body against your leg and protect the head from injury. Stay with the resident; do not move him or her, and call for assistance. Report the details to your supervisor and assist with completing an incident report.

Passive Range of Motion Exercises

1. Raise the bed to a comfortable working height and lock the wheels.

2. Position the resident in the supine position with pillow under head.

3. Exercise each shoulder, rotating the shoulder joint smoothly; abduct and adduct the shoulder.

4. Supporting the wrist and elbow, exercise the elbow and forearm by flexing and extending the lower arm.

5. Rotate and flex the wrists, one wrist at a time, from side to side (ulnar deviation and radial deviation).

6. Flex and extend each hand at the wrist.

7. Flex and extend the fingers and thumb of each hand.

8. Exercising each leg at a time, support the foot from behind the ankles, and flex the lower legs by bending the knee.

9. Throughout movements, ask resident about pain. If the resident experiences pain at any point in the procedures, stop at that point and report the resident's pain and its location to the nurse.

10. Exercising each leg at a time, support each foot from behind the ankles, and adduct and abduct the legs at the hip.

11. Exercising each hip at a time, rotate each leg at the hip, supporting the ankle.

12. Supporting each foot behind the instep, rotate, flex, and extend the foot at the ankle.

13. Grasp, flex, and extend the toes.

> **CAUTION**
>
> If the resident complains of sudden pain in the calf when performing steps 11 or 12, stop the procedure and notify the nurse because this could be a symptom of a blood clot in the lower leg.

Monitoring Resident in Restraints

Follow facility policy on frequency of checking on resident status while in restraints as well as removal schedule. Failure to follow policy could be considered negligence.

Provide comfort for resident while in restraints.

Feeding

1. Follow agency policy for proper identification of the resident to ensure that the meal is the correct one prepared for the resident.

2. Position resident in sitting position.

3. Offer and assist resident to toilet and/or wash hands before feeding.

4. Sit at eye level with resident for feeding.

5. Protect clothing from spills.

6. Provide fluids (at least every 3 to 4 bites of food) to drink during feeding. Encourage the resident to choose which food to eat next throughout the feeding.

7. Use a spoon to feed resident.

8. Make sure resident has swallowed before offering additional bites of food.

9. Encourage resident to complete meal to receive maximum benefit of diet.

10. Talk with resident during feeding to encourage interaction and increase satisfaction with feeding experience.

11. Leave area around resident's mouth clean and dry.

12. Record food intake in percentages.

13. Document I & O for fluids as ordered for the resident.

14. Report any resident problems with feeding procedure.

Offering the Bedpan

1. To protect bed linens, place a protective pad directly under resident's buttocks.

2. Using the correct size bedpan to fit the resident (a fracture pan might be necessary for immobilized resident), ask the resident to roll to opposite or position resident on side opposite you and place the bedpan under resident to allow for comfort and collection of urine or stool.

3. After the bedpan is in place, raise the head of bed to resident's comfort level.

4. Provide resident with toilet tissue before removing the bedpan.

5. Before removing the bedpan, lower the head of the bed. Anchor the bedpan firmly as the resident rolls away from it.

6. Empty bedpan contents into toilet.

7. Cleanse and dry the perineal area as necessary to remove urine or stool.

8. Rinse, dry, and store bedpan in bottom drawer of bedside cabinet.

9. Record output (record total urine output in cc or mL, according to facility procedure; if recording stool, estimate the amount expelled).

10. Report unusual amount, color, odor, and consistency of stool or resident discomfort.

Performing Ostomy Care

1. Carefully remove ostomy appliance that is attached to the skin.

2. Gently but firmly cleanse the skin around the stoma with soap and water, and dry the area thoroughly.

3. Apply skin protector around the stoma as ordered.

4. Empty the collection bag and note the amount, color, and consistency of the stool.

5. Wash thoroughly with soap and water.

6. Reattach the appliance per manufacturer's instructions and fasten the clamp to prevent leakage.

7. Record the procedure and report any redness, irritation, open lesions, or resident discomfort to the nurse.

Administering a Cleansing Enema

1. Assemble equipment and supplies at the bedside; prepare the cleansing enema solution: Keep water temperature at 105°F; add manufacturer's soap to water (do not use bar soap); flush enema tubing with water to expel air from tubing; clamp tubing securely.

2. Raise the side rails and raise the bed to a comfortable working position.

3. Assist the resident onto the left side in the Sim's position and cover with a bath blanket.

4. Position an I.V. pole beside the bed and raise the side rail.

5. Hang the enema bag on I.V. pole with the tubing at the bottom of the bag. Hang no higher than 18 inches above the bed or 12 inches above the resident's anus.

6. Apply gloves.

7. Lower the side rail and place a protective pad under the resident's buttocks.

8. Lubricate four inches of the tip of the enema tubing.

9. Ask the resident to breathe deeply to help relieve cramping during the procedure.

10. With one hand, lift the upper buttock to expose the anus; with other hand, carefully insert the tubing tip into the rectum, rotating it approximately 2–4 inches into the rectum. If you feel resistance or the resident complains of pain, stop the procedure and notify the nurse.

11. Unclamp the tubing and allow the solution to flow slowly into the rectum. If the resident complains of cramping, clamp the tubing and stop the flow; resume in a minute or so to instill as much liquid as possible.

12. Ask the resident to hold the solution inside the rectum as long as possible.

13. Lower the bed position and assist the resident to the bathroom or the bedside commode; if unable to leave the bed, place the resident on a bedpan to expel the enema fluid and stool; place the call light within easy reach.

14. Discard the equipment and supplies in the garbage receptacle and clean area.

15. Return to the bedside or bathroom when the resident has completed the toileting process.

16. Provide perineal care.

17. Observe the expelled stool; flush toilet or empty commode or bedpan.

18. Apply clean gloves; wash and disinfect commode or bedpan and return for storage; remove gloves and wash hands.

19. Lower the bed and raise the side rails per facility policy.

20. Record the amount, color, and consistency of the expelled stool.

Recording Intake and Output (I & O)

1. Identify foods considered to be liquid and estimate intake by the resident.

2. Record amount of liquid taken by the resident in cubic centimeters (cc) or milliliters (mL), according to facility policy.

3. Measure output by pouring the contents of the urine receptacle (urinal or bedpan) into a graduate. Place graduate on a clean barrier and on a flat surface to read the amount of urine at eye level.

4. Flush the urine down the toilet.

5. Rinse and disinfect the graduate and bedpan or urinal according to facility policy. Remove gloves.

6. Using a pen, record the amount of urine in the Output column of the I & O form.

7. Report any unusual color, amount, odor, or particles noted in the urine to the nurse.

Measuring and Recording Output from a Urinary Drainage Bag

1. With gloved hands, open drain (at bottom of urinary drainage bag) and drain the urine into the graduate, which is placed on a barrier of two paper towels on the floor. Empty urine bag into graduate without touching drain to the graduate.

2. Wipe drain with alcohol swab after emptying urine and return drain to the cover on the urinary drainage bag, being careful not to touch the drain to the bag while inserting it into the cover.

3. Secure urinary drainage bag to the bed frame; never hang the bag on the side rail or other movable part of the bed.

4. Place graduate at eye level on a flat surface covered with a paper towel to read the level of urine collected.

5. Empty urine into toilet; rinse and store the graduate; discard the paper towel.

6. Remove gloves and wash hands.

7. Record output.

8. Report any unusual odor, color, consistency, or particles noted in the urine to your supervisor.

Indwelling Catheter Care

1. Raise the resident's bed to a comfortable working height. Provide for privacy by screening the resident from view.

2. Position the resident: For a female, position dorsal recumbent (on back) with head slightly elevated and knees bent; for a male, use the supine or Fowler's position.

3. Place waterproof pad under resident's buttocks.

4. Cover resident to expose only the perineal area.

5. For a female, use your non-dominant hand to gently pull open labia to fully expose urethral meatus and catheter insertion site, keeping hand in this position throughout procedure. For a male, use your nondominant hand to retract the foreskin if not circumcised, and hold penis firmly at shaft just below the glans (end of penis), keeping hand in this position throughout the procedure.

6. Observe urethral meatus and tissue for color, odor, swelling, and consistency of discharge.

7. Cleanse perineal tissue: keep water in bath basin at temperature that is 110 to 115 degrees. Check periodically throughout the procedure to assure water temp is comfortable for the resident.

8. For a female, one clean, soapy cloth and cleanse urethral meatus toward anus and catheter, from top of meatus toward anus. Use only one cloth per wipe. Do *not* return dirty cloth to clean water. For a male, while spreading urethral meatus, cleanse around catheter first, then wipe in circular motion around meatus and glans to base of the penis. Rinse area with warm, clean water, one cloth per wipe. Dry well.

9. While holding the catheter with your nondominant hand, cleanse down the catheter 3 to 4 inches. Rinse and blot area and catheter dry with clean towel.

10. For uncircumcised male residents, replace the foreskin over the glans.

11. Remove the pad from under the buttocks and leave the resident on a dry pad.

12. Check tubing. Observe tubing for proper drainage, keeping tubing free of kinks or obstructions. Assure that the resident is not lying on drainage tubing.

13. Keep drainage bag lower than the bladder; assure that the bag is attached to the bed frame, *not* the bed side rail and not on the floor.

14. Position resident for comfort.

15. Unscreen the resident.

16. Dispose of equipment, making sure the bath basin is washed and dried before storing.

17. Report and record characteristics of drainage, appearance of perineal area, or any discomfort reported by the resident.

Applying a Condom Catheter

1. Provide perineal care.

2. Remove the protective backing from the catheter's adhesive surface.

3. Roll the catheter onto the penis, moving from the end of the penis (glans) toward the body.

4. Leave one inch of space between the penis and the end of the catheter.

5. Apply tape in spiral direction to secure the catheter. Never completely encircle the penis (to avoid a tourniquet effect).

6. Connect the catheter to the drainage bag.

7. Tape the catheter to the resident's inside thigh to prevent traction on the catheter.

8. Fasten the drainage bag to the bed frame. Never fasten the drainage bag to a movable part of the bed.

9. Record the procedure and the resident's response.

10. Remove the catheter for perineal care at least once daily; report any redness, swelling, or discomfort to the nurse.

11. Add the specimen amount to the output total.

Collecting Specimens

Prepare specimen label and follow the procedures for the different specimens documented in the sections that follow.

SAFETY TIP

All specimens should be placed in a laboratory biohazard bag, sealed and stored, or transported to the laboratory according to agency policy.

Routine Urine Specimen

1. Assisting if necessary, ask the resident to urinate into a clean bedpan, urinal, or specimen collection pan (*hat*).

2. Carefully remove the specimen container lid and lay the lid on a solid surface with the inside up.

3. Pour at least 5ccs (mLs) of urine from the bedpan, urinal, or hat into the specimen container.

4. Carefully replace the lid on the container to avoid touching the inside of the lid or the container.

5. Clean and store the bedpan or urinal in the bottom drawer of the bedside table; never place the urinal or the bedpan on the overbed table.

6. Attach the label to the container and take the container to the designated location.

Clean Catch Urine Specimen

1. Provide perineal care.

2. Position the resident on a bedpan, provide a urinal, or assist to the bathroom.

3. Carefully remove the specimen container lid and lay the container lid on a solid surface with the inside up.

4. Instruct the resident to begin voiding and then stop.

5. Holding the specimen container under the resident, instruct him or her to resume voiding and collect at least 5ccs of urine.

6. Instruct the resident to finish voiding.

7. Carefully replace the lid on the container to avoid touching the inside of the lid or the container.

8. Clean and store the bedpan or urinal in the bottom drawer of the bedside table; never place the urinal, bedpan, or hat on the overbed table.

9. Attach the label to the container and take the container to the designated location.

Urine Specimen from an Indwelling Catheter

CNAs do not collect urine specimens from an indwelling catheter because this is a sterile procedure reserved for the nurse.

Stool Specimen

1. Assist the resident to void if necessary.

2. Carefully remove the specimen container lid and lay the container on a solid surface with the inside up.

3. Place the resident on a bedpan or place a specimen pan (hat) under the toilet seat.

4. Instruct the resident not to dispose of toilet tissues into the bedpan or hat; provide a disposable bag for soiled tissues.

5. Place the call light within easy reach.

6. When the resident is finished, remove the resident from the bedpan or assist from the bathroom.

7. Provide perineal care.

8. With gloved hands, use a tongue depressor to transfer one to two tablespoons of stool from the bedpan to the specimen container.

9. Wrap the tongue depressor in paper towel and discard it in the disposable bag.

10. Remove gloves; carefully replace the lid on the container to avoid touching the inside of the lid or the container.

11. Clean and store the bedpan in the bottom drawer of the bedside table; never place the bedpan on the overbed table.

12. Place the disposable bag of tissues in a biohazard waste container.

13. Attach the label to the container and take the container to the designated location.

14. Add the stool elimination to the daily stool count.

Isolation Procedures

Isolation procedures follow CDC guidelines for various medical conditions that require protection among residents to control the spread of disease. The following guidelines apply to individual supplies and equipment that might be required for a particular type of isolation.

Choking Relief

When discovering a resident who is choking and loses consciousness:

1. Ease the resident to the floor; attempt respirations.

2. If breath will not enter, reposition the resident to help expose the airway; attempt respirations again.

3. If still unsuccessful, use firm back slaps, chest thrusts, abdominal thrusts until the object is dislodged and can be removed.

4. After removing the object, check for pulse and respirations. If neither is present, start chest compressions and/or rescue breathing until the resident resumes breathing or until relieved by another rescuer.

Putting on Disposable Gown, Gloves, Goggles, and Mask

1. Remove watch and place on a paper towel for transport into resident room (keep on towel until needed for vital signs).

2. Wash hands and dry thoroughly.

3. Put on disposable gown with opening at the back; tie the neck ties.

4. Tie the gown's waist ties, ensuring that the back edges of the gown cover your uniform.

5. Don a mask, adjusting it to cover your nose and mouth; tie the mask securely at the back of your head or slip elastic bands on the side of the mask over your ears.

6. Don goggles over eyes and adjust to fit well.

7. Don gloves, ensuring that the gown cuffs are covered by the cuff edges of the gloves.

Removing Disposable Gown, Gloves, Goggles, and Mask

1. Remove gloves, turning them inside out and placing them in the biohazardous waste receptacle.

2. Wash hands.

3. Holding them only by the elastic bands, remove goggles or face shield.

4. Without touching the outside of the gown, ease one hand inside the cuff of the gown on the opposite arm and pull the gown down over the other arm.

5. Using the same technique, pull the gown down from the other arm.

6. Fold and roll the gown away from you, with outside (contaminated side) folded to the inside.

7. Discard the gown in the biohazardous waste receptacle.

8. Remove the mask by grasping only the ties or elastic bands at the mask sides.

9. Untie the bottom tie first, and then the top tie or slip the elastic bands over your ears.

10. Dispose of the mask in a covered trash receptacle.

11. Wash and dry your hands.

12. Place your watch in your pocket; dispose of the paper towel in the trash receptacle.

13. Use a paper towel to open the door of the resident's room.

14. Discard the towel inside the room.

15. Repeat handwashing per facility policy.

Assisting with Post-Mortem Care

1. Wash hands.

2. Collect the following:

   ▶ Post-mortem kit, containing shroud/body bag

   ▶ Bed linen protector

   ▶ Towels and washcloths

   ▶ Bath basin

   ▶ Denture cup

   ▶ Tape

   ▶ Cotton balls

   ▶ Valuables envelope

3. Don gloves.

4. Raise bed and adjust to flat position to promote good body mechanics.

5. Place body in supine position.

6. Gently place the eyelids over the eyes. Apply moistened cotton balls over each eye if needed to keep eyes closed.

7. Follow agency policy regarding denture care. In most cases, leave in place and notify the nurse so he/she can record that dentures are in the resident's mouth.

8. Close the resident's mouth (you may place a rolled washcloth beneath the chin to maintain alignment).

9. Follow agency policy for jewelry removal. Record all jewelry removed.

10. Unless an autopsy is ordered, assist the nurse to remove all drainage bags, tubes, and catheters.

NOTE

To avoid contamination, follow aseptic technique in dispose of soiled dressings, linens, and other resident care items.

11. Wash body with plain water and dry thoroughly.

12. Replace soiled dressings with clean ones.

13. Dress body in a clean gown.

14. Comb hair and rearrange as needed.

15. Use tags and identify the body (apply to ankle and opposite big toe).

16. Place body in shroud and label outside of the shroud.

17. Cover the body with a clean sheet up to shoulder level.

18. Label all gathered resident belongings. Leave the labeled denture cup with the body.

19. Tidy up the room.

20. Remove gloves and wash hands.

21. Pull the privacy curtain and close the resident's room door.

22. Per agency procedure, discard used supplies and return equipment to area for cleaning.

23. Following agency procedure, report disposition (what was done) with resident's valuables.

Practice Exam I

This exam consists of 75 questions that reflect the material covered in this book. The questions are representative of the types of questions you should expect to see on the Certified Nursing Assistant Examination; however, they are not intended to match exactly what is on the exam.

Some of the questions require that you decide on the best possible answer. Often, you are asked to identify the best course of action to take in a given situation. Read the questions carefully and thoroughly before you attempt to answer them. For best results, treat this exam as if it were the actual examination. When you take it, time yourself, read carefully, and answer all the questions to the best of your ability.

The answers to all the questions appear in "Answers to Practice Exam 1." Check your letter answers against those in the answer key, and then read the explanations provided. You might also want to return to the chapters in the book to review the material associated with any questions you have answered incorrectly. Also, review the tables in Appendix A, "Nursing Assistant Test Cross-Reference," which maps the questions to the nine categories of questions that you will encounter on the written exam, as listed by the National Nurse Aide Assessment Program (NNAPP):

▶ Member of health-care team

▶ Activities of daily living

▶ Client rights

▶ Basic nursing skills

▶ Emotional and mental health needs

▶ Communication

▶ Restorative skills

▶ Spiritual and cultural issues

▶ Legal and ethical behavior

Exam Questions

1. Where is the best location for the physical therapist to stand when ambulating a resident who has experienced a stroke?

   ○ **A.** On the resident's affected side

   ○ **B.** Behind the resident

   ○ **C.** On the resident's unaffected side

   ○ **D.** In front of the resident

2. What is the best action for the nursing assistant caring for a resident who is agitated and talking loudly?

   ○ **A.** Tell the resident he or she needs to be quiet because he or she is disturbing the other residents.

   ○ **B.** Speak to the resident in a calm and comforting manner.

   ○ **C.** Ask to have your assignment changed.

   ○ **D.** Report the behavior to the nurse.

3. Gloves are worn to protect residents when the nursing assistant performs which of the following activities?

   ○ **A.** Changing the resident's clothes

   ○ **B.** Feeding the resident

   ○ **C.** Performing peri-care

   ○ **D.** Changing the resident's position in the chair

4. Which statement best describes the term *neglect*?

   ○ **A.** Changing the resident as soon as you discover he or she is soiled

   ○ **B.** Leaving the floor after reporting to your supervisor

   ○ **C.** Calling for assistance when needed to care for the resident

   ○ **D.** Applying a restraint too tight

5. When a resident is dying, what sense is generally lost last?

   ○ **A.** Taste

   ○ **B.** Smell

   ○ **C.** Hearing

   ○ **D.** Sight

6. What is the first sign of a decubitus ulcer developing on a resident's skin?

    ○ **A.** Bleeding

    ○ **B.** Redness

    ○ **C.** Bruising

    ○ **D.** Swelling

7. In which of the following activities does the nursing assistant demonstrate correct listening skills?

    ○ **A.** Speaking at the same time as the resident

    ○ **B.** Leaning toward the resident and responding when appropriate

    ○ **C.** Talking to the resident while continuing to work

    ○ **D.** Asking the right questions to lead the direction of the conversation

8. In which location is the body temperature of a resident taken most often?

    ○ **A.** Oral

    ○ **B.** Rectal

    ○ **C.** Axillary

    ○ **D.** Tympanic

9. What is the important basic procedure for the nursing assist to perform to increase muscle strength and joint mobility of a resident who is unable to voluntarily move his or her limbs?

    ○ **A.** Resistance exercises

    ○ **B.** Aerobic exercises

    ○ **C.** Active range of motion exercises

    ○ **D.** Passive range of motion exercises

10. Where is the best position for the nursing assistant to stand when assisting a resident to transfer to a wheelchair?

    ○ **A.** Left side of the wheelchair

    ○ **B.** Right side of the wheelchair

    ○ **C.** In front of the wheelchair

    ○ **D.** Behind the wheelchair

11. What is the first step a nursing assistant should take when performing a procedure?

    ○ **A.** Informing the nurse that you are going to the resident's room to perform the procedure

    ○ **B.** Checking the resident's identification

    ○ **C.** Providing privacy

    ○ **D.** Documenting the procedure

12. Which muscles are injured most often when a nursing assistant does not use proper body mechanics?

  ○ **A.** Back muscles

  ○ **B.** Shoulder muscles

  ○ **C.** Neck muscles

  ○ **D.** Leg muscles

13. All the following are the safety precautions used for showering a resident, except

  ○ **A.** Checking the water temperature before assisting the resident into the shower

  ○ **B.** Locking the wheels on the shower chair

  ○ **C.** Leaving the resident unattended in the shower

  ○ **D.** Promptly drying and covering the resident after the shower is completed

14. Which phrase best defines the term STAT?

  ○ **A.** As soon as possible

  ○ **B.** Within the next 2 to 3 hours

  ○ **C.** By the end of the shift

  ○ **D.** Immediately

15. What is the most appropriate action of the nursing assistant when a resident complains of chest pain?

  ○ **A.** Provide the resident with water

  ○ **B.** Place the resident in prone position

  ○ **C.** Call for help immediately

  ○ **D.** Check the resident's blood sugar

16. A bed that is free of wrinkles is necessary to prevent which of the following complications?

  ○ **A.** Pressure sore

  ○ **B.** Agitation

  ○ **C.** Hypertension

  ○ **D.** Infection

17. The dietitian shared with the nursing assistant that vitamin D is found in which of the following foods?

  ○ **A.** Bread and cereals

  ○ **B.** Fruits and vegetables

  ○ **C.** Protein

  ○ **D.** Dairy

18. Which statement is true regarding the rights of a resident's religious beliefs?

  ○ **A.** Employees are to impose their religious beliefs on the residents.

  ○ **B.** Employees are never to discuss religious beliefs with residents.

  ○ **C.** Residents have a right to practice their own religious beliefs.

  ○ **D.** Family members are responsible to bring the religious leaders in to speak to the residents.

19. What is the best way to improve communication with a resident who is 100% deaf?

  ○ **A.** An amplified phone system

  ○ **B.** A loud voice

  ○ **C.** Reduced noise

  ○ **D.** Pen and paper

20. What is the main purpose of restorative (rehabilitation) care?

  ○ **A.** To help the patient return to work or home

  ○ **B.** To live as independently and safely as possible

  ○ **C.** To teach the resident to care for self

  ○ **D.** To aid in the healing process

21. What is the illegal activity a nursing assistant can be charged with when they threaten to restrain a resident?

  ○ **A.** Assault

  ○ **B.** Battery

  ○ **C.** Slander

  ○ **D.** Negligence

22. Select the appropriate equipment to use when giving mouth care to an unconscious resident.

   ○ **A.** Toothbrush

   ○ **B.** Toothpaste

   ○ **C.** Mouthwash

   ○ **D.** Soft toothette

23. Where is a resident's radial pulse located?

   ○ **A.** Ankle

   ○ **B.** Foot

   ○ **C.** Wrist

   ○ **D.** Groin

24. Which of the following is the medical term for intestinal gas?

   ○ **A.** Feces

   ○ **B.** Flatus

   ○ **C.** Flank

   ○ **D.** Friction

25. What statement suggests an understanding by the nursing assistant of cultural awareness?

   ○ **A.** All cultures are the same.

   ○ **B.** Once a person enters this country, he or she should learn the culture.

   ○ **C.** Care is planned to include a resident's cultural needs.

   ○ **D.** Culture does not influence the care of residents.

26. Which of the following best defines quadriplegia?

   ○ **A.** Flaccid lower extremities

   ○ **B.** No movement of all four extremities

   ○ **C.** Inability to move the left side

   ○ **D.** No feeling of both feet

27. How can a nursing assistant encourage the independence of a resident when assisting with a.m. (morning) care?

    ○ **A.** Allowing the resident to do as much as possible for himself or herself and then assisting with the rest of the a.m. care

    ○ **B.** Waiting until the resident is well rested and then offering a.m. care

    ○ **C.** Providing the resident with the needed materials and then leaving him or her alone to complete the a.m. care without further assistance

    ○ **D.** Waiting until the resident complains of the need to be cleaned, and then he or she will want to do more for himself or herself

28. It is appropriate for the nursing assistant to share resident information with all of the following persons, except

    ○ **A.** The physician caring for the resident

    ○ **B.** A member of the resident's church

    ○ **C.** The nurse caring for the resident

    ○ **D.** The nursing assistant who will be caring for the resident

29. When assisting a resident who has right-sided weakness to get dressed in the morning, which arm is placed in the sleeve of the shirt first?

    ○ **A.** Right side (the affected side)

    ○ **B.** Left side (the non-affected side)

    ○ **C.** Both sides at the same time

    ○ **D.** Whichever side is easiest for the nursing assistant

30. What product is applied to a resident's skin before shaving?

    ○ **A.** Shaving cream

    ○ **B.** Alcohol

    ○ **C.** Cold water

    ○ **D.** Lotion

31. A resident has just been told of a family member's death. The best way to help the resident deal with the death is by which of the following actions?

    ○ **A.** Assuring him or her that everyone eventually dies

    ○ **B.** Allowing him or her to grieve alone

    ○ **C.** Sharing with him or her that the family member is in a better place

    ○ **D.** Staying with the resident and encouraging him or her to talk.

32. When can a nursing assistant refuse to do a delegated task?

   ○ **A.** When the task is not part of the nursing assignment's assignment

   ○ **B.** When it is not a task a nursing assistant should perform

   ○ **C.** When the nursing assistant has completed the task once this shift

   ○ **D.** When the nurse is sitting at the desk talking to other nurses

33. What is the last action taken by a nursing assistant when making a resident's bed?

   ○ **A.** Handwashing

   ○ **B.** Removing all wrinkles from the bed

   ○ **C.** Repositioning the bed to a low position

   ○ **D.** Placing the call light near the resident

34. Which of the following is the correct definition for NPO?

   ○ **A.** Nothing by mouth

   ○ **B.** Only liquids by mouth

   ○ **C.** Resident may only have ice chips

   ○ **D.** Resident may have only thickened liquids

35. Who is responsible to ask visitors to leave the resident's room before giving the resident a bath?

   ○ **A.** The charge nurse

   ○ **B.** Someone in housekeeping

   ○ **C.** The nursing assistant preparing to give the bath

   ○ **D.** The nurse assigned to the resident

36. The following statements are correct regarding the resident's phone rights, except

   ○ **A.** Telephones are provided to each resident.

   ○ **B.** Access to phones and privacy is provided to each resident.

   ○ **C.** Telephones can be used under supervision.

   ○ **D.** Resident access is provided during daytime hours only.

37. According to Elizabeth Kübler-Ross, the first stage of grief is

   ○ **A.** Denial

   ○ **B.** Acceptance

   ○ **C.** Anger

   ○ **D.** Bargaining

38. Select the best definition for restorative nursing.

    ○ **A.** Helping to regain strength

    ○ **B.** Promoting well-being

    ○ **C.** Increasing self-care ability

    ○ **D.** All of the above

39. Who should the nursing assistant report to when the resident is threatening to leave the facility without physician permission?

    ○ **A.** Physician

    ○ **B.** Supervisor

    ○ **C.** Nurse

    ○ **D.** Dietician

40. Which of the following is least likely to cause a skin tear?

    ○ **A.** Ring or watch

    ○ **B.** Friction

    ○ **C.** Short cropped nails

    ○ **D.** Pulling on an extremity

41. A fellow nursing assistant comes to work under the influence of marijuana. As a member of the health-care team, what is the best action of the nursing assistant?

    ○ **A.** Inform the nurse immediately.

    ○ **B.** Ignore it.

    ○ **C.** Tell the nursing assistant to get help.

    ○ **D.** Give the nursing assistant coffee to drink.

42. An assigned resident does not want lifesaving measures to be performed if he expires. The term the nursing assistant would find written on the chart is

    ○ **A.** NPO

    ○ **B.** DNR

    ○ **C.** CPR

    ○ **D.** ADL

43. The entire foot needs to be watched for breaks in the skin. What area of the foot is most often overlooked?

   ○ **A.** The heel

   ○ **B.** The bottom of the feet

   ○ **C.** Between the toes

   ○ **D.** Balls of the foot

44. What should a nursing assistant do when he or she recognizes that a resident is not eating enough?

   ○ **A.** Offer dietary supplements as prescribed.

   ○ **B.** Administer vitamins to the resident.

   ○ **C.** Provide an additional tray.

   ○ **D.** Tell the nurse.

45. When a resident falls, what is the most frequent injury that occurs?

   ○ **A.** Broken wrist

   ○ **B.** Fractured ankle

   ○ **C.** Strained ligament

   ○ **D.** Fractured hip

46. For what condition would the nursing assistant be directed by the nurse to apply a cold pack?

   ○ **A.** To decrease a burn injury

   ○ **B.** To stop bleeding

   ○ **C.** To decrease swelling

   ○ **D.** To stop back pain

47. The nursing assistant recognizes which of the following is not a sign of impending death?

   ○ **A.** Decreased respirations

   ○ **B.** Irregular, weak, and thready pulse

   ○ **C.** Skin cool and moist

   ○ **D.** Stable vital signs

48. Select the observation that should be reported to the nurse STAT?

- ○ **A.** Cloudy yellow urine
- ○ **B.** Brown loose stools
- ○ **C.** Respiratory rate of 38
- ○ **D.** Radial pulse of 80

49. The resident is to be placed in Fowler's position. Select the correct description of this position.

- ○ **A.** Head of bed 45 to 60 degrees with legs either bent or straight
- ○ **B.** Head of bed flat
- ○ **C.** Bed flat with feet higher than the head
- ○ **D.** Head of bed 15 degrees with legs either bent or straight

50. When helping to lift a resident up in bed, which of the following positions demonstrates proper use of body mechanics?

- ○ **A.** Keep your back and knees straight, and lift using your thigh muscles.
- ○ **B.** Bend slightly at the waist, keep knees partially flexed, and lift with your legs muscles.
- ○ **C.** Bend slightly at the waist, keep knees partially flexed, and lift with your back muscles.
- ○ **D.** Use whatever position and muscles make you feel most comfortable.

51. Washing your hands appropriately is important to reduce the spread of infection. All of the following directions are correct regarding hand washing, except

- ○ **A.** Rub hands vigorously with soap and water for at least 30 seconds.
- ○ **B.** Use a clean paper towel to dry hands.
- ○ **C.** If hands are visibly soiled, you may use an alcohol-based hand sanitizer.
- ○ **D.** Use paper towel to turn off faucet.

52. In order for gloves to provide adequate protection, the nursing assistant must remember to do which of following?

- ○ **A.** Wash your hands before and after glove use.
- ○ **B.** Wash your hands after taking off gloves only.
- ○ **C.** A small tear will still keep out germs.
- ○ **D.** Always wear latex gloves because they are less costly.

53. It is important for the nursing assistant who is caring for a resident who is anxious to do which of the following?

   ◯ **A.** Have restraints available in case of escalation to violence.

   ◯ **B.** Remain calm and speak softly.

   ◯ **C.** Keep the room bright.

   ◯ **D.** Turn on the television to distract the resident.

54. When a confused resident is placed in restraints by the nurse, the nursing assistant knows which of the following is true?

   ◯ **A.** The resident should not be touched because the resident might cause harm to others.

   ◯ **B.** The resident is being punished.

   ◯ **C.** Assessment of the resident needs such as bathroom, repositioning, and circulation must be conducted at least every 2 hours.

   ◯ **D.** Residents are not allowed to have any visitors.

55. After you have finished washing the resident's feet, look at the patient and their surrounds for safety problems. One example of a safety problem that requires immediate attention is which of the following?

   ◯ **A.** Bed in low position and head of the bed elevated

   ◯ **B.** Wet area on the floor next to the bed

   ◯ **C.** Bedside table within the resident's reach

   ◯ **D.** Call light within reach of the patient

56. The nursing assistant is walking a resident around the unit, and the resident starts to fall. The first action of the nursing assistant should be which of the following?

   ◯ **A.** Leave the resident and quickly grab the nearest chair.

   ◯ **B.** Get behind the resident and ease the patient to ground slowly.

   ◯ **C.** Get to the nearest phone and call for assistance.

   ◯ **D.** Grab the resident by the arms and lift him or her up.

57. Which is the definition of a resident who becomes more confused each day during evening hours or after dark?

   ◯ **A.** Alzheimer's disease

   ◯ **B.** Dementia

   ◯ **C.** Psychosis

   ◯ **D.** Sundowner's Syndrome

58. What is the correct action by the nursing assistant to provide emotional support for a resident when assisting the resident with a shower?

  ○ **A.** Make sure the door is closed to the shower room.

  ○ **B.** Talk about your weekend activities with the other nursing assistants.

  ○ **C.** Be sure to call the resident by his or her first name.

  ○ **D.** Check the water temperature before beginning the shower.

59. A nursing assistant smells smoke in the nursing facility. A resident is found smoking a cigarette in his or her room. What is the correct action of the nursing assistant?

  ○ **A.** Tell the resident to be more careful so no one catches him or her.

  ○ **B.** Tell the resident that it is against the law and to go outside.

  ○ **C.** Tell the resident that it is a safety hazard and ask him or her to go outside.

  ○ **D.** Do nothing as long as the resident isn't bothering anyone.

60. The resident consumed 3 ounces of juice. How many milliliters should the nursing assistant document on the flow sheet?

  ○ **A.** 120mL

  ○ **B.** 60mL

  ○ **C.** 45mL

  ○ **D.** 90mL

61. When the CNA washes a resident's feet, the water temperature should be

  ○ **A.** Hot

  ○ **B.** Tepid

  ○ **C.** Cold

  ○ **D.** Warm

62. What is the nursing assistant's appropriate response to a resident who is making sexual comments?

  ○ **A.** "Thank you, no one has flirted with me in a long time."

  ○ **B.** "I am going to ignore that comment."

  ○ **C.** "The comment is not acceptable to me."

  ○ **D.** "I bet you tell all the girls that."

63. What device is used to prevent contractures?

   ◯ **A.** Hand roll

   ◯ **B.** Cane

   ◯ **C.** Back support

   ◯ **D.** Ace bandage

64. What is the medical term for high blood pressure?

   ◯ **A.** Tachycardia

   ◯ **B.** Hypertension

   ◯ **C.** Bradypnea

   ◯ **D.** Hypotension

65. It is important for residents to be provided oral care daily to prevent one of the following problems:

   ◯ **A.** Oral infections

   ◯ **B.** Stomach disorders

   ◯ **C.** Bowel problems

   ◯ **D.** Tooth breakage

66. Which of the following is the correct method of washing the perineum of a resident who has an indwelling catheter?

   ◯ **A.** Wash from the rectum to the meatus.

   ◯ **B.** Wash the meatus with peroxide.

   ◯ **C.** Wash away from the meatus.

   ◯ **D.** Provide traction to the catheter while washing the meatus.

67. The nursing assistant is cleaning a resident's dentures. What is the correct safety precaution?

   ◯ **A.** The nursing assistant places a towel in the sink while cleaning the dentures.

   ◯ **B.** The nursing assistant keeps the dentures in a glass on the sink to soak.

   ◯ **C.** The nursing assistant places the dentures on the bedside table for easy access.

   ◯ **D.** The nursing assistant places the dentures on tissues in the sink while cleaning the dentures.

68. The resident calls the nursing assistant into his room to tell her that his dentures are lost. What is the best action for the nursing assistant to take first?

    ⭕ **A.** Tell the resident that he will be able to eat without them because he is on a pureed diet.

    ⭕ **B.** Notify the charge nurse.

    ⭕ **C.** Go through all the resident's belongings in case he hid them.

    ⭕ **D.** Notify the resident's family.

69. The nursing assistant overhears a conversation about a resident on the elevator at work. The nursing assistant knows this is a violation of which patient right?

    ⭕ **A.** The resident's right to be present when his care is discussed

    ⭕ **B.** The resident's right to refute any statements made

    ⭕ **C.** The resident's right to privacy

    ⭕ **D.** The resident's right to medical care

70. Washing your hands as a nursing assistant is very important. Which of the following is a part of the handwashing procedure?

    ⭕ **A.** Drying both hands thoroughly with a discarded towel

    ⭕ **B.** Applying soap to both hands before turning on the water

    ⭕ **C.** Applying friction for at least 20 seconds

    ⭕ **D.** Wiping soiled hands on a towel as the first step in the procedure

71. What is the correct procedure when using a gait belt?

    ⭕ **A.** Use a rocking and pulling motion when using the belt to get up from a sitting position.

    ⭕ **B.** Stand on the resident's strong side.

    ⭕ **C.** Two or more caregivers are needed when using a gait belt.

    ⭕ **D.** Proper body mechanics are not needed with use of a gait belt.

72. Which of the following is the correct method for counting respirations?

    ⭕ **A.** Look at your watch and the resident's abdomen at the same time.

    ⭕ **B.** Look at your watch, count 10 respirations, and then examine your watch again.

    ⭕ **C.** Look only at the abdomen and count to 30.

    ⭕ **D.** Look at your watch and have a second nursing assistant count the respirations.

73. When providing oral care to the unconscious or conscious resident, the CNA should brush all the following areas except:

   ○ **A.** Teeth

   ○ **B.** Gums

   ○ **C.** Lips

   ○ **D.** Tongue

74. One of the residents you care for is a member of your church. When someone from the church inquires about the resident's medical condition, your best response should be:

   ○ **A.** Inform the person that all information regarding all residents is confidential, and you cannot disclose the information to him or her.

   ○ **B.** Tell the person that the resident's condition is unchanged and that he or she should visit the resident soon.

   ○ **C.** Ignore the request for the information and talk about upcoming church activities.

   ○ **D.** Tell the person to ask the resident's nurse for information.

75. When the CNA washes a patient's hair, the best way to keep it from tangling and matting is to

   ○ **A.** Trim the hair.

   ○ **B.** Wash and condition hair daily.

   ○ **C.** Brush or comb hair daily.

   ○ **D.** Place hats on the patient's head in between washes.

Answers to Practice Exam I

Answers at a Glance

1. A	26. B	51. C
2. B	27. A	52. A
3. C	28. B	53. B
4. D	29. A	54. C
5. C	30. A	55. B
6. B	31. D	56. B
7. B	32. B	57. D
8. A	33. A	58. A
9. D	34. A	59. C
10. C	35. C	60. D
11. B	36. B	61. D
12. A	37. A	62. C
13. C	38. D	63. A
14. D	39. C	64. B
15. C	40. C	65. A
16. A	41. A	66. C
17. D	42. B	67. A
18. C	43. C	68. B
19. D	44. D	69. C
20. B	45. D	70. C
21. A	46. C	71. A
22. D	47. D	72. A
23. C	48. C	73. C
24. B	49. A	74. A
25. C	50. B	75. C

Rationales for Answers to Practice Exam I

1. **A.** When assisting a resident who has had a stroke to ambulate, the nursing assistant stands on the affected side to support the resident. Standing behind the resident (B), on the resident's strong side (C), or in front of the resident (D) does not provide the support the resident requires.

2. **B.** Speaking in a calm comforting manner is appropriate communication for an agitated resident. Telling the resident to be quiet (A), asking to have your assignment changed (C), and reporting the behavior to the nurse (D) are all negative forms of communication; they will either increase agitation or avoid communication with the resident.

3. **C.** With peri-care the nursing assistant has a greater chance of coming into contact with blood or body fluids. When changing the resident's clothes (A), feeding the resident (B), and changing the resident's position in the chair (D), there is less chance of contaminations.

4. **D.** Applying a restraint too tight might cause injury to the resident and is considered neglect. Changing the resident as soon as you discover he or she is soiled (A), leaving the floor after reporting to your supervisor (B), and calling for assistance when needed to care for the resident (C) are appropriate care of the resident.

5. **C.** Hearing is the last sense lost before dying. It is important for family members to know that the resident might not be able to communicate, but he or she might still hear them talking. A resident might lose his or her senses of taste (A), smell (B), or sight (D); however, those senses are typically lost before hearing when the resident is dying.

6. **B.** One of the first signs of a pressure sore is redness, then blanching, and after that skin breakdown. Bleeding (A) is a late sign that occurs after the skin is broken. Bruising (C) and swelling (D) are not signs of a pressure sore, but of trauma to the area.

7. **B.** Sitting, leaning in, and making eye contact are forms of effective communication. Speaking at the same time as the resident (A), talking to the resident while continuing to work (C), and making sure to ask the right questions to lead the direction of the conversation (D) are ways that might stop the resident from communicating with the nursing assistant.

8. **A.** Oral temperature is the route most often obtained due to access. Rectal (B), axillary (C), and tympanic (D) are routes that are used when the resident is mouth breathing or cannot hold the thermometer in his or her mouth.

9. **D.** Passive range of motion exercises are performed to increase or maintain muscle movement in residents who cannot move the muscles on their own. Resistance exercises (A), aerobic exercises (B), and active range of motion exercises (C) are examples of exercises that require the resident to be alert and actively participating.

10. **C.** The nursing assistant stands in front of the wheelchair as he or she pivots the resident into the wheelchair. Standing on the left side of the wheelchair (A), right side of the wheelchair (B), or behind the wheelchair (D) does not provide the support the resident needs for the transfer to the wheelchair and could cause the resident to fall.

11. **B.** The first step before performing a procedure is to identify the resident. Informing the nurse that you are going to the resident's room to perform the procedure (A), providing privacy (C), and documenting the procedure (D) are correct actions, but they are not the first step before performing a procedure.

12. **A.** The back muscles are injured most often when proper body mechanics are not adhered to. The shoulder muscles (B), neck muscles (C), and leg muscles (D) can be injured when a nursing assistant does not use proper body mechanics for a procedure, but not as often as the lower back muscles.

13. **C.** Leaving the resident unattended in the shower might cause the resident harm. Choices A, B, and D are all part of the procedure for showering a resident. Check the water temperature to prevent scalding (A). Lock the shower chair to help prevent the resident from a fall injury (B). Dry and cover the resident to aid in the prevention of the resident chilling and provide privacy (D).

14. **D.** STAT means the activity needs to be carried out immediately. The order for STAT is used when there is an emergency or when harm to the resident is threatened. As soon as possible (A), within the next 2 to 3 hours (B), and by the end of the shift (C) are not quick enough to be consider STAT.

15. **C.** Chest pain has many serious causes, and the resident needs immediate attention. Providing the resident with water (A) is incorrect because the resident should be kept NPO until the nurse informs the nursing assistant that the resident can have fluids. Placing the resident in prone position (B) is an inappropriate position for a resident with chest pain. Checking the resident's blood sugar (D) is a diagnostic test ordered by the physician or at the determination of the nurse.

16. **A.** To prevent a pressure sore, the resident's linen needs to be wrinkle free along with turning the resident frequently and changing the resident quickly when he or she becomes soiled. Agitation (B), hypertension (C), and infection (D) are not a result of wrinkled linen.

17. **D.** Vitamin D is found in dairy products. Bread and cereals are from the whole grains and cereal group (A), fruits and vegetables are from the fruits and vegetables group (B), and protein is from the protein group (C).

18. **C.** According to the Resident's Bill of Rights, the resident is to be able to practice his or her beliefs. The resident, not the family, has the right to request the facility to contact a religious leader who will contact the resident (D). Employees who impose their religious beliefs (A) or discuss religious beliefs with the residents (B) are both a violation of the resident's rights.

19. **D.** When someone is completely deaf (hearing no sound), the only form of communication from the offered options might be lip reading or pen and paper. Communicating with an amplified phone system (A), a loud voice (B), or in a reduced noise environment (C) are good forms of communication for someone who is not completely deaf but has a percentage of deafness.

20. **B.** The main purpose of restorative (rehabilitation) care is to assist the person to live as independently and safely as possible. A, C, or D are incorrect because the resident may not be able to return to home or work, to care for self, or to improve healing even with restorative plan of care.

21. **A.** Threatening harm is assault. Battery is actual harm to a resident (B). Slander is malicious verbal defamation of someone's character (C). Negligence is causing harm to someone from neglect of duties or responsibility (D).

22. **D.** Soft toothettes are used with an unconscious resident to lessen the chance of aspiration of fluid and toothpaste into the lungs. Toothbrush (A) and toothpaste (B) are used with the conscious resident or with the cleaning of dentures. Mouthwash is harsh and might be aspirated (C).

23. **C.** The radial pulse is located on the wrist. The tibialis posterior (A) is located on the ankle, the pedal pulse is on the foot (B), and the femoral pulse is found in the groin area (D).

24. **B.** Flatus is the medical term for intestinal gas. Feces is the term used for stool (A). Flank is the term used to describe the side of the back (C). Friction is a means of tension to an area by the force from another source (D).

25. **C.** Culture influences the resident's choices in food, clothing, and lifestyle. Many cultures have similarities but still are unique, suggesting choice A is incorrect. Residents have rights to live without feeling they are being treated unfairly due to their culture, so choice B is incorrect. Culture might influence almost every area of care, making choice D incorrect.

26. **B.** A person who is a quadriplegic is paralyzed in all four limbs. Answer A is known as a paraplegic. Inability to move one side is generally due to a stroke (C), and no sensation in the feet is known as neuropathy (D).

27. **A.** Promoting independence is to encourage the resident to do as much for himself or herself as possible and then assist with the rest. Waiting until the resident is well rested and then offering a.m. care (B) is partially correct because the resident who is rested might be able to complete more of his or her self-care. C and D are incorrect because they could be considered a form of negligence.

28. **B.** Only those who are caring for the resident are to have access to information about the resident. The physician, nurse, and nursing assistant (A, C, and D) all have a right to access the records of the resident.

29. **A.** The nursing assistant is to assist the person on the weak side to provide support and help to prevent the resident from falling. Choices B, C, and D are all incorrect.

30. **A.** Shaving cream softens the beard without drying the skin. Alcohol (B) dries the skin and may cause a burning sensation, and cold water (C) does not soften the beard. Lotion used with shaving might irritate the skin (D).

31. **D.** Sitting quietly with the resident and listening when he or she wants to share something about the loved one is the best source of comfort. Responses A, B, and C do not allow the resident to feel free to talk about the loved one.

32. **B.** The nursing assistant should only refuse to complete a delegated task when it is not part of the nursing assistant's duties, such as giving a medication for the nurse. Responses A, C, and D do not describe scenarios where the nursing assistant has a legal obligation or should refuse to complete a delegated task.

33. **A.** Handwashing is the last action of nursing assistants. Removing all wrinkles from the bed (B), repositioning the bed into a low position (C), and fastening the call light near the resident (D) are all a part of the procedure, but are performed before the final act of handwashing.

34. **A.** NPO is the medical term for nothing by mouth, the withholding all food and fluids. The resident might be NPO for a procedure or surgery in the morning. The statements, only liquids by mouth, ice chips, and thickened liquids (answers B, C, and D) are incorrect.

35. C. One of the nursing assistant's duties is to ensure client privacy at all times. Asking the family to leave the room is intended to provide adequate privacy. The charge nurse (A), someone in housekeeping (B), and the nurse assigned to the resident (C) are not responsible.

36. B. The resident has a right to access phones and privacy to make phone calls as requested. Although the resident has a right to phone access, having a phone for each resident is not part of the resident's rights (A). Telephone use under supervision only (C) and phone access during daytime hours only (D) restrict the resident's right to phone use.

37. A. According to the stages of grief by Elizabeth Kübler-Ross, denial is the first stage. Choices B, C, and D are each a stage that a resident might go through, but they are not the first stage.

38. D. Restorative nursing is helping the resident regain strength, promoting well-being, and increasing his or her ability to care for himself or herself.

39. C. The nurse needs to be notified immediately when a resident is threatening to leave the facility against medical advice (AMA). The nurse, not the nursing assistant, notifies the physician, supervisor, and dietician (A, B, and D).

40. C. Fingernails of the nursing assistant should be kept clean and short to protect residents from scratches or tears to the skin. A ring or watch (A), friction (B), or pulling on an extremity (D) could cause the skin of an elderly resident to tear.

41. A. An impaired employee is more likely to be involved in an injury to self or a resident. If you are aware of anyone working who is impaired and you do not report it, you could also be held responsible for a staff member's or resident's injury. Selections B, C, and D all involve hiding the impairment from the employer.

42. B. DNR is the medical abbreviation used for "do not resuscitate." If the resident stops breathing or does not have a pulse, he or she does not want CPR or other forms of lifesaving measures to be performed. NPO is the medical abbreviation for non per os, which means nothing by mouth (A). CPR is the medical abbreviation for cardiopulmonary resuscitation (C). ADL is the medical abbreviation for activities of daily living (D).

43. C. When examining and cleaning the feet, the area most overlooked is the between the toes. When the areas are not dried well or become dried, the skin breaks down. The heel (A), the bottom of the feet (B), and the balls of feet (D) are seldom overlooked because they are easy visible.

44. D. Telling (reporting) to the nurse an important change, such as not eating, is one of the roles of the nursing assistant. (A) Many of the residents have a form of dietary liquid drink ordered by the physician when they are not receiving enough calories, but they should not be given it without first checking with the nurse. Administering vitamins to the resident (B) is considered administration of a medication and is out of the scope of the nursing assistant's role. Providing an additional tray of food is inappropriate if the resident did not eat the first tray (C).

45. D. The hip is a common site for a fracture when a resident falls. Although a broken wrist (A), fractured ankle (B), or strained ligament (C) could occur during a fall, they are not considered common sites for injury when a resident falls.

46. C. Cold application is used to decrease swelling. Burn injuries require moist dressings (A). Pressure is used to stop bleeding (B). Heat is used to decrease back pain (D).

47. **D.** When a person is dying, you do not typically see stable vital signs. The blood pressure drops to below normal; the respirations become shallow (A); the pulse becomes irregular, weak, and thready; and the skin becomes moist and cool (C).

48. **C.** A respiratory rate of 38 is abnormal and might indicate the resident is in severe respiratory distress. Cloudy yellow urine (A), brown loose stools (B), and a radial pulse of 80 (D) need to be reported to the nurse but not immediately.

49. **A.** Fowler's position is the head of the bed raised at least 45 degrees with the legs bent or straight. Head of the bed flat (B) describes supine position. Bed flat with feet higher than the head (C) describes trendelenburg position. Head of bed 15 degrees with legs either bent or straight (D) describes supine position with head of the bed slightly raised.

50. **B.** The correct position for the nursing assistant when lifting a resident up in bed is to slightly bend the waist, slightly flex the knees, and use his or her leg muscles. The choices in responses A, C, and D do not protect the nursing assistant from injury.

51. **C.** When hands are visibly soiled, they must be washed with soap and water. Hand sanitizer can be used when they are not visibly soiled. Rubbing hands vigorously with soap and water for at least 30 seconds (A), using a clean paper towel to dry hands (B), and using a paper towel to turn off the faucet (D) are all correct steps in washing your hands.

52. **A.** Hands are washed before and after glove use. Washing hands after taking off gloves only (B) and assuming that a small tear will still keep out germs (C) are incorrect uses of gloves and might increase chances of contamination. Always wearing latex gloves because they are less costly (D) is incorrect because the nursing assistant or the resident might be allergic to latex.

53. **B.** Remaining calm and speaking softly helps to reduce the tension in the room. Having restraints available in case of escalation to violence (A), keeping the room bright (C), and turning on the television to distract the resident (D) increase or aggravate the resident's anxiousness.

54. **C.** Residents who are in restraints are offered food, fluids, and toileting assistance at least every two hours. Selections A, B, and D are examples of isolation or forms of punishment. Restraints are not to be used for punishment but to prevent the resident from harming himself or herself.

55. **B.** A wet area on the floor could be a potential hazard for the resident and the staff. Responses A, C, and D are positive activities that protect the resident from harm.

56. **B.** Easing the resident onto the ground decreases or prevents the chance of injury to the resident and the nursing assistant. Leaving the resident and quickly grabbing the nearest chair (A), getting to the nearest phone and calling for assistance (C), grabbing the resident by the arms and lifting the resident up (D) might cause harm to the resident.

57. **D.** Residents who are more confused at night or during evening hours is referred to as Sundowner's Syndrome. Alzheimer's disease (A) and dementia (B) are disorders that cause decreased orientation, but are not related to nighttime. Psychosis (C) is a psychiatric condition that presents with decreased orientation and is not related to a specific time of day.

58. **A.** One way to provide emotional support is to provide privacy by closing the door to the shower room. Choice B excludes the resident choice. Choice C is disrespectful, and choice D is important and will provide comfort but not security.

59. C. Smoking inside a building where oxygen is in use is a hazard, and residents might have conditions where smoke causes harm. Telling the resident to be more careful so no one catches him or her (A) or doing nothing (D) are ignoring the facility's policies and putting other residents in harm's way. Telling the resident that smoking in the building is against the law and to go outside (B) is only partially correct.

60. D. There are 30 milliliters in each ounce, so 3 ounces is equivalent to 90 milliliters. Choices A, B, and C are incorrect.

61. D. To provide comfort for the patient and not harm, the water should be warm. Selections A, B, and C are incorrect. Cold water can cause pain. Hot water can burn the resident, and tepid water is uncomfortable.

62. C. Whenever a sexual comment is made, the first step is to set boundaries and let the resident know the comment or action is not acceptable. It is also advisable to report the incident to the nurse caring for the resident. Choices A and D might encourage further comments or actions. Choice B focuses on the resident and not the resident's behavior.

63. A. A hand roll is used to prevent contracture to the hand of a resident who is unconscious or has paralysis to the extremity. A cane (B), back support (C), and Ace bandage (D) are assistive or support devices.

64. B. Hypertension is the medical term for high blood pressure. Tachycardia (A) is the term for increased pulse rate. Bradypnea (C) is the term for decreased respiratory rate. Hypotension (D) is the term for low blood pressure.

65. A. The main reason to provide oral care is to prevent oral infections. Selections B, C, and D are conditions that can occur from long-term dental and gum disease.

66. C. Washing of the perineum when a resident has an indwelling catheter includes washing from the meatus to the labia to prevent the introduction of bacteria that might be present on the catheter into the urinary tract. Washing from the rectum to the meatus (A) introduces bacteria to the urinary system. Washing the meatus with peroxide (B) is incorrect because peroxide is not a cleanser. Providing traction to the catheter while washing the meatus (D) causes unnecessary discomfort to the resident.

67. A. Dentures are expensive and difficult to replace, and loss will cause stress to the resident. Use precaution when cleaning wet dentures by padding the sink so that dentures are less likely to break if the teeth are dropped accidently. Keeping the dentures in a glass (B), placing them on the bedside table (C), or placing them on tissue paper in the sink while washing (D) does not adequately protect the dentures.

68. B. Report all lost items to the charge nurse as soon as possible. Telling the resident to eat without his or her dentures (A) or going through the resident's belongings to see whether they are hidden (C) are not respectful of the client or his or her belongings. Notifying the resident's family of the loss (D) is the responsibility of the facility administrator.

69. C. Confidentiality is the right of the resident, so care should not be discussed on an elevator where other people can overhear. The resident's right to be present when his or her care is discussed (A), the resident's right to refute any statements made (B), and the resident's right to medical care (D) are all rights of the resident, but do not apply to this situation.

70. **C.** When washing hands, friction for at least 20 seconds is needed to remove soil and germs. Selection A is incorrect because a clean towel should be used to dry hands. Choice B is incorrect; soap is applied after the water is turned on, and soil is to be rinsed from the hands, not placed on a dry towel, making choice D incorrect.

71. **A.** A rocking and pulling motion on the belt is used to lift the resident from the chair to a standing position. Standing on the resident's strong side (B) is the wrong choice because the nursing assistant needs to stand on the resident's weak side and place the chair or wheelchair on the resident's strong side. The need for more than one caregiver (C) is not required in the use of the gait belt, which is used to provide additional support for the resident and the nursing assistant. Proper body mechanics should be used at all times to prevent injury, so answer D is incorrect.

72. **A.** The procedure calls for the nursing assistant to look at her watch and count respirations in a 30-second to 1-minute interval. The choices in choices B, C, and D lead to inaccurate data.

73. **C.** Toothbrushes are abrasive and should not be used on the lips. Choices A, B, and D are the correct areas to brush when assisting the resident to brush his or her teeth.

74. **A.** Only persons who are directly caring for residents have a right to information regarding the resident. Telling the person that the resident's condition is unchanged and that he or she should visit the resident soon (B) gives information about the resident's condition and is a break in confidentiality. Ignoring the request for the information and discussing upcoming church activities (C) and telling the person to ask the resident's nurse if they need any information (D) are incorrect responses.

75. **C.** To keep the hair from tangling and knotting, it is important to brush and /or comb the hair daily. Choice A is incorrect; the resident or family members care for trimming and styling of the hair. Choice B is not practical and may dry the resident's hair. Choice D is incorrect because it is the resident's choice to wear a hat or other accessories.

Practice Exam II

This exam consists of 75 questions that reflect the material covered in this book. The questions are representative of the types of questions you should expect to see on the Certified Nursing Assistant Examination; however, they are not intended to match exactly what is on the exam.

Some of the questions require that you deduce the best possible answer. Often, you are asked to identify the best course of action to take in a given situation. Read the questions carefully and thoroughly before you attempt to answer them. For best results, treat this exam as if it were the actual examination. When you take it, time yourself, read carefully, and answer all the questions to the best of your ability.

The answers to all the questions appear in "Answers to Practice Exam II." Check your letter answers against those in the answer key, and then read the explanations provided. You might also want to return to the appropriate chapters in the book to review the material associated with any questions you have answered incorrectly. Also, review the tables in Appendix A, "Nursing Assistant Test Cross-Reference," which maps the questions in the nine different categories of questions that you will see on the written exam as listed by the National Nurse Aide Assessment Program:

- ▶ Member of health-care team
- ▶ Activities of daily living
- ▶ Client rights
- ▶ Basic nursing skills
- ▶ Emotional and mental health needs
- ▶ Communication
- ▶ Restorative skills
- ▶ Spiritual and cultural issues
- ▶ Legal and ethical behavior

Exam Questions

1. Which of the following is the recommended position for a resident in order to obtain his or her blood pressure?

   ○ **A.** Lying with feet elevated

   ○ **B.** Sitting with both feet on the floor

   ○ **C.** Standing, with arms at the resident's side

   ○ **D.** Lying flat

2. When a resident requests to pray before a procedure, what is the optimum response of the nursing assistant?

   ○ **A.** Allow the resident privacy to pray.

   ○ **B.** Ask the resident to pray silently while you perform the procedure.

   ○ **C.** Explain to the resident that the procedure needs to be completed now and that praying will need to wait.

   ○ **D.** Tell the resident you have already prayed for him or her this morning and now it is time to perform the procedure.

3. How frequently should the nursing assistant record the totaled intake and output in the resident's chart?

   ○ **A.** After each meal

   ○ **B.** Every six hours

   ○ **C.** At the end of the shift

   ○ **D.** Every four hours

4. What is the medical term for low blood pressure?

   ○ **A.** Tachycardia

   ○ **B.** Hypertension

   ○ **C.** Bradypnea

   ○ **D.** Hypotension

5. How often should the nursing assistant turn a resident who is unable to move himself or herself?

   ○ **A.** Every three hours

   ○ **B.** Every two hours

   ○ **C.** Every four hours

   ○ **D.** At least once a shift

6. Which condition is expected in an older resident?

   ○ **A.** Slowing of responses

   ○ **B.** Inability to make decisions

   ○ **C.** Increased agitation

   ○ **D.** Loss of long-term memory

7. When the nursing assistant is helping a resident to shave, he or she should remember to do which of the following?

   ○ **A.** Use shaving cream to soften the hair.

   ○ **B.** Wash the resident's face and then dry the skin thoroughly before shaving.

   ○ **C.** Shave in the opposite direction of hair growth with a sharp razor.

   ○ **D.** Apply alcohol after shaving to keep the skin clean.

8. A CNA confirms a patient received his or her correct diet by which of the following?

   ○ **A.** Matching the resident's food tray/diet items with resident's diet order

   ○ **B.** Checking for the patient's likes and dislikes

   ○ **C.** Sitting the resident in an upright position

   ○ **D.** Weighing the food before and after the resident eats.

9. What is the normal range of a resident's pulse at rest?

   ○ **A.** 55–105 beats per minute

   ○ **B.** 60–100 beats per minute

   ○ **C.** 45–65 beats per minute

   ○ **D.** 70–120 beats per minute

10. A resident is scheduled for a procedure and is NPO. What type of tray would be delivered to the resident?

   ○ **A.** A can of Sprite and frozen treat

   ○ **B.** Salad and cottage cheese

   ○ **C.** No tray will be delivered

   ○ **D.** Applesauce and toast

11. Which type of device would the physician order to help a resident with ambulation?

   ○ **A.** Orthodontic

   ○ **B.** Feeding

   ○ **C.** Transfer

   ○ **D.** Assistive

12. Of the statements that follow, which is not an example of the Patient's Bill of Rights?

   ○ **A.** Right to privacy and dignity

   ○ **B.** Right of confidentiality

   ○ **C.** Right to accept or refuse treatment

   ○ **D.** Right to mistreat staff and fellow residents

13. An alcohol-based hand cleanser should not be considered in which of the following situations?

   ○ **A.** After contact with a resident

   ○ **B.** When soap and water are not available

   ○ **C.** When hands are visibly soiled

   ○ **D.** After assisting a resident to the shower

14. Which definition that follows describes sensory impairment?

   ○ **A.** Inability to read

   ○ **B.** Inability to use a bike

   ○ **C.** Loss of hearing

   ○ **D.** Inability to write

15. What activity by the CNA will increase a resident's feeling of safety?

   ○ **A.** Checking the resident's identification before any activity or procedure

   ○ **B.** Calling the resident "honey" or "dear"

   ○ **C.** Leaving the resident unattended during elimination

   ○ **D.** Informing the resident to yell out if he or she needs help

16. A nursing assistant can help meet the resident's spiritual needs by which of the following?

   ○ **A.** Telling the resident about his or her beliefs

   ○ **B.** Letting the resident know that the resident is not to talk about his or her beliefs

   ○ **C.** Allowing the resident to share his or her beliefs

   ○ **D.** Inviting someone from your church to talk to the resident

17. While trimming a resident's nails, you accidently cut his or her finger. This is considered which of the following legal terms?

   ○ **A.** Physical abuse

   ○ **B.** Negligence

   ○ **C.** Malpractice

   ○ **D.** Assault

18. What is the initial step before feeding a resident?

   ○ **A.** Informing the kitchen staff of what type of diet the patient wants

   ○ **B.** Assisting the resident in washing his or her hands and face

   ○ **C.** Checking the resident's chart to see what type of diet the patient is ordered

   ○ **D.** Making sure the resident eats all of his or her main meal before serving dessert

19. The first action of a nursing assistant who discovers a fire is to do what?

   ○ **A.** Rescue the patient

   ○ **B.** Pull the fire alarm

   ○ **C.** Extinguish the fire

   ○ **D.** Follow the evacuation plan

20. A nursing assistant's false report to the charge nurse that another nursing assistant accepted a tip from a resident is an example of which of the following?

   ○ **A.** Negligence

   ○ **B.** Defamation

   ○ **C.** Malpractice

   ○ **D.** Insubordination

21. What measurement is used when documenting a resident's intake and output?

   ○ **A.** Ounces

   ○ **B.** Milligrams

   ○ **C.** Milliliters

   ○ **D.** Cups

22. The nursing assistant notices mail for a resident at the nurse's station. The correct action of the nursing assistant is which of the following?

   ○ **A.** Discard the resident's junk mail.

   ○ **B.** Open the mail for the resident.

   ○ **C.** Deliver the mail unopened to the resident's room.

   ○ **D.** Give the mail to a family member.

23. What is the best course of action when taking the oral temperature of a resident who just finished drinking a glass of iced tea?

- ○ **A.** Wait approximately 15 minutes.
- ○ **B.** Go ahead and take the oral temperature.
- ○ **C.** Wait approximately 45 minutes.
- ○ **D.** Skip the temperature now and take it the next scheduled time.

24. If linen drops on the floor while making a resident's bed, the CNA's next action would be to:

- ○ **A.** Pick up the linen, shake it out, and use it.
- ○ **B.** Place the linen on the bedside chair to use at a later time.
- ○ **C.** Leave the linen on the floor for housekeeping to pick up.
- ○ **D.** Place the linen in the hamper because it is soiled.

25. Which of the following is a safety device used to move a resident from the bed to the chair?

- ○ **A.** Hoyer lift
- ○ **B.** Slide board
- ○ **C.** Brace
- ○ **D.** Assistive

26. The Patient's Bill of Rights is a document that lists the guidelines concerning the resident's treatment, level of care, and services received while in the facility. Any complaints or dissatisfaction by the resident in regard to care is called what?

- ○ **A.** Slander
- ○ **B.** Defamation
- ○ **C.** Irritating
- ○ **D.** Grievance

27. Select the appropriate action by the nursing assistant that demonstrates adherence to the resident's right to privacy.

- ○ **A.** When assisting the resident onto the bedside commode, the nursing assistant forgets to close the curtains.
- ○ **B.** While the resident is talking on the phone, the nursing assistant stands beside the resident.
- ○ **C.** Before beginning a procedure, the nursing assistant closes the curtains.
- ○ **D.** When dressing the resident, the nursing assistant does not provide adequate clothing.

28. Seizures are also known as:

　　○　**A.** Sugar in the blood

　　○　**B.** Convulsions

　　○　**C.** Consumption

　　○　**D.** Heart troubles

29. Select the appropriate medical term for the abnormal shortening of muscle tissue.

　　○　**A.** Arthritis

　　○　**B.** Sprain

　　○　**C.** Fracture

　　○　**D.** Contracture

30. Which of the following is not the responsibility of the nursing assistant when caring for a resident who is receiving intravenous therapy?

　　○　**A.** Watching the site for swelling, redness, or bruising

　　○　**B.** Monitoring the site, tubing, and infusion solution

　　○　**C.** The CNA does not have any responsibility for the infusion.

　　○　**D.** Watching the flow infusion and then communicating any problems

31. What complication should be reported immediately to the nurse?

　　○　**A.** Incontinence

　　○　**B.** Difficulty breathing

　　○　**C.** Weak leg

　　○　**D.** Increased hunger

32. Select the appropriate action of the nursing assistant when a resident refuses to transfer out of the bed into the chair.

　　○　**A.** Threaten the resident if he or she continues to refuse.

　　○　**B.** Ignore the resident and transfer him or her anyway.

　　○　**C.** Call for help to transfer the resident because he or she might become agitated.

　　○　**D.** Respect the resident's wishes.

33. Of the following signs, which one is not a sign of infection?

　　○　**A.** Fever

　　○　**B.** Swelling

　　○　**C.** Redness

　　○　**D.** Shortness of breath

34. The resident reports eliminating a black and sticky stool. The best action of the CNA is which of the following?

- ○ **A.** Tell the resident to call the next time he or she has a stool so you can verify what he or she is reporting.
- ○ **B.** Report what the resident told you to the nurse.
- ○ **C.** Visualize the rectum to see if any stool is present.
- ○ **D.** Tell the resident that the stool is probably related to what he or she ate for breakfast.

35. Residents might experience which of the following due to decreased intestinal motility?

- ○ **A.** Liquid stools
- ○ **B.** Increased stools
- ○ **C.** Constipation
- ○ **D.** Increased appetite

36. What is the best use of restraints?

- ○ **A.** To protect the resident from harm
- ○ **B.** As a punishment
- ○ **C.** To decrease time spent attending to the resident
- ○ **D.** To keep the resident out of the way

37. Who is the best source of information regarding the history of the resident upon his or her admission?

- ○ **A.** A friend
- ○ **B.** A family member
- ○ **C.** The physician
- ○ **D.** The resident

38. What is the correct action when washing your hands?

- ○ **A.** Apply soap before wetting your hands.
- ○ **B.** Keep hands elevated above your waist.
- ○ **C.** Apply friction for 5 seconds.
- ○ **D.** Use a clean, dry paper towel to turn off the water.

39. Select the appropriate location for a thermometer when taking an axillary temperature.

   ○ **A.** Place the probe of the thermometer 1 inch under the arm.

   ○ **B.** Place the probe in the posterior 1/3 of the axillia.

   ○ **C.** Place the probe of the thermometer in the center of the axilla.

   ○ **D.** Place the probe in the anterior 1/3 of the axillia.

40. Which of the following is *not* a step in attaining a radial pulse?

   ○ **A.** Place the fat pads of your finger over the groove in the wrist.

   ○ **B.** Use a watch with a second hand or one with a digital readout for the procedure.

   ○ **C.** Lightly press against the radial bone.

   ○ **D.** To obtain the pulse rate, count the beat for 10 secs and then multiply by 6.

41. The nursing assistant is preparing to assist a resident with a partial bath. Which action is appropriate?

   ○ **A.** Use only tepid water.

   ○ **B.** Cover the resident with a towel.

   ○ **C.** Close the curtain to provide privacy.

   ○ **D.** Wash the feet first.

42. Which of these statements regarding nail care is false?

   ○ **A.** Dry the resident's hands and feet after soaking.

   ○ **B.** Report any breaks in the skin to the nurse.

   ○ **C.** Soak hands and feet at a safe temperature.

   ○ **D.** Rub lotion between the toes to prevent skin from breaking.

43. What is the appropriate container for storing dentures?

   ○ **A.** A denture cup filled with water

   ○ **B.** Several wet paper towels

   ○ **C.** A large jar filled with mouthwash

   ○ **D.** The drawer of the bedside table

44. The definition of the center of rehabilitative care is:

   ○ **A.** To improve the resident's capabilities

   ○ **B.** To restore function to as near normal as possible

   ○ **C.** To return the resident to better than normal functioning

   ○ **D.** To prevent harm and injury

45. Restorative nursing is best described as:

   ○ **A.** Focusing on doing things for the residents

   ○ **B.** Creating long-range goals with the resident

   ○ **C.** Preventing deterioration when possible

   ○ **D.** Assisting the resident in remembering his or her limitations

46. Which statement about taking a rectal temperature is true?

   ○ **A.** The electronic thermometers do not need lubrication.

   ○ **B.** Only mercury thermometers provide an accurate temperature.

   ○ **C.** The normal rectal temperature is 1 degree lower than an oral temperature.

   ○ **D.** Privacy is provided during the procedure.

47. Which radial pulse should you repeat?

   ○ **A.** 88 beats per minute and regular

   ○ **B.** 59 beats per minute and irregular

   ○ **C.** 60 beats per minute and regular

   ○ **D.** 96 beats per minute and regular

48. Which of the following actions regarding the CPR procedure for one rescuer is false?

   ○ **A.** Wait to start CPR until help arrives.

   ○ **B.** Call for help and activate the emergency response system.

   ○ **C.** Get the AED.

   ○ **D.** Look for breathing.

49. When one of the residents is in restraints, what is the responsibility of the nursing assistant?

   ○ **A.** Apply tape securely around the mitt restraints to keep them fastened.

   ○ **B.** Check extremities for circulation, motion, and sensitivity over a 4-hour period.

   ○ **C.** Document the reason for application of restraints in the chart.

   ○ **D.** Promote resident comfort throughout the use of restraints.

50. Which statement by the nursing assistant best reflects appropriate communication?

   ○ **A.** "What can I do about your life situation?"

   ○ **B.** "Rest awhile and you will feel better in the morning."

   ○ **C.** "I can't help you right now; I am busy."

   ○ **D.** "I can see this bothers you. I will convey your concerns to the nurse."

51. Which finding should be reported to the nurse immediately when the resident is using splints for ambulation?

    ○ **A.** Sweating

    ○ **B.** Refusing to use the splint

    ○ **C.** Difficulty in application

    ○ **D.** Pain with use

52. The nursing assistant should use a mask when entering the room of a resident who has been placed on what type of precautions?

    ○ **A.** MRSA precautions

    ○ **B.** Droplet precautions

    ○ **C.** Contact precautions

    ○ **D.** Standard precautions

53. Which action is used by the nursing assistant when caring for a resident with a condom catheter?

    ○ **A.** Pull the catheter onto the penis.

    ○ **B.** Remove the catheter at least once daily and report any problems.

    ○ **C.** Ensure that the catheter is well lubricated.

    ○ **D.** Attach the drainage bag to the side rail.

54. Which health-care team member is responsible for locating resources to manage resident care?

    ○ **A.** Nurse

    ○ **B.** Social Worker

    ○ **C.** Nurse Assistant

    ○ **D.** Physician

55. Which action would the nursing assistant carry out when assisting a resident to use the bedpan?

    ○ **A.** Protect the bed with an absorbent pad.

    ○ **B.** Raise the head of the bed and then roll the resident to his or her side.

    ○ **C.** Use the fracture pan on everyone.

    ○ **D.** Leave the bedpan in the bed after use.

56. All of the following are the correct care of a resident with a beard, except

    ○ **A.** Wash the beard daily.

    ○ **B.** Trim the beard daily.

    ○ **C.** Comb the beard daily.

    ○ **D.** Wash the beard when it is visibly soiled.

57. Which of the following would the nursing assistant not chart as input?

- ○ **A.** Ice cream for snack
- ○ **B.** Soup at lunch
- ○ **C.** Intravenous fluids
- ○ **D.** Jell-O at night

58. What should the nursing assistant report immediately after the resident has received an enema?

- ○ **A.** Severe abdominal cramping
- ○ **B.** Expelled brown liquid
- ○ **C.** Increased amount of flatus
- ○ **D.** Large amount of formed feces

59. Why is an indwelling catheter taped or secured to the resident's leg?

- ○ **A.** To ensure the catheter does not fall out
- ○ **B.** To prevent trauma to the resident
- ○ **C.** To allow the resident to use the bathroom if needed
- ○ **D.** To prevent leaking around the catheter

60. Which of the following health-care team members is responsible for carrying out the medical plan under the supervision of the Registered Nurse?

- ○ **A.** Physician
- ○ **B.** Nursing Assistant
- ○ **C.** Licensed Practical Nurse
- ○ **D.** Physical Therapist

61. The nursing assistant is walking down the hall with an armful of supplies and notices a spill on the floor. Which of the following is the correct action of the nursing assistant?

- ○ **A.** Walk by and say nothing.
- ○ **B.** Stop at the nurse's station and tell whoever is there about the spill.
- ○ **C.** Tell the first person you see to have housekeeping come by and clean up the spill.
- ○ **D.** Put down the supplies and clean up the spill immediately.

62. A resident you are assigned has an ostomy drainage bag that is scheduled to be changed. What is your first action?

  - ○ **A.** Apply skin protector around the stoma.
  - ○ **B.** Empty the collection bag.
  - ○ **C.** Cleanse around the stoma gently with soap and water.
  - ○ **D.** Reattach the clean bag to the apparatus around the stoma.

63. What should the CNA do if he or she accidently cuts the resident while shaving him or her?

  - ○ **A.** Apply pressure to the cut.
  - ○ **B.** Apply a band aid to the cut.
  - ○ **C.** Apply tissue paper to the cut.
  - ○ **D.** Apply shaving lotion to the cut.

64. A resident is exhibiting signs of depression. Which of the following is not a sign of depression?

  - ○ **A.** Loss of appetite
  - ○ **B.** Increased sleeping
  - ○ **C.** Increased interest in activities
  - ○ **D.** Crying

65. A resident who has discovered he or she is dying is crying a lot. What should the nursing assistant do?

  - ○ **A.** Ignore the resident as much as possible.
  - ○ **B.** Tell the resident to begin to live each day to the fullest.
  - ○ **C.** Stay with the resident as much as possible.
  - ○ **D.** Explain to the resident that he or she might not die for awhile yet.

66. A resident is receiving oxygen therapy through a nasal cannula. When should the nasal cannula be removed?

  - ○ **A.** Every hour
  - ○ **B.** Every 2 hours
  - ○ **C.** Every 8 hours
  - ○ **D.** Long enough to clean the nose

67. A resident whose spouse has recently died cries frequently. What should the nursing assistant do?

- ○ **A.** Change the subject.
- ○ **B.** Introduce him or her to the other available residents on the unit.
- ○ **C.** Stay and listen to the resident as much as possible.
- ○ **D.** Tell the resident that things will get better over time.

68. While cleaning a resident's dentures, the CNA accidently drops one and it breaks. What is the CNA's best course of action?

- ○ **A.** Report the accident to the resident and the nurse.
- ○ **B.** Show the resident the dentures and ask him or her what happened to them.
- ○ **C.** Hide the dentures.
- ○ **D.** Offer to pay for the broken denture.

69. The resident is wearing an elastic bandage on her arm, and the CNA notices swelling and discoloration of the skin. What should the CNA do?

- ○ **A.** Complete the resident's a.m. care and then report the swelling and discoloration to the nurse.
- ○ **B.** Elevate the arm.
- ○ **C.** Report the swelling and discoloration to the nurse immediately.
- ○ **D.** Remove the elastic bandage.

70. Which of the following is not a healthy way for a nursing assistant to reduce stress in his or her life?

- ○ **A.** Get plenty of rest and eat a balanced diet.
- ○ **B.** Get involved in a new hobby.
- ○ **C.** Go out several times a week for drinks after work.
- ○ **D.** Exercise several times a week.

71. If a resident's family becomes angry at the nursing assistant, what action should the nursing assistant take?

- ○ **A.** Tell the family member it is not your fault.
- ○ **B.** Quickly walk away.
- ○ **C.** Tell them you do not have to stand for this behavior.
- ○ **D.** Stay calm and inform the nurse caring for the resident.

72. The CNA can encourage a resident's rehabilitation by which of the following?

- ○ **A.** Doing everything for the resident for a few days until he or she feels comfortable at the rehab facility
- ○ **B.** Showing sympathy for the resident's situation
- ○ **C.** Not talking about the activities the resident cannot do by himself or herself
- ○ **D.** Focusing on what the resident can do for himself or herself

73. A nursing assistant is overheard telling a resident that the nurse caring for her is not a good nurse. The nursing assistant could be charged with which of the following?

- ○ **A.** Slander
- ○ **B.** Malpractice
- ○ **C.** Negligence
- ○ **D.** Assault

74. A resident is dying and requests the CNA to stay with him or her because he or she is afraid. The best action of the CNA is to

- ○ **A.** Ask the nurse if the resident can have a sleeping pill because he or she cannot sleep.
- ○ **B.** Stay with the resident and let him or her share his or her feelings and concerns.
- ○ **C.** Tell the resident you will call his or her family for him or her.
- ○ **D.** Call the doctor.

75. Elastic stockings are applied to the resident's legs to help reduce venous stasis. Which of the following is a critical step to remember with the application and monitoring?

- ○ **A.** Pull the stocking up smoothly over the legs.
- ○ **B.** Make sure that the stockings are wrinkle free at all times.
- ○ **C.** Support the resident's foot at the heel.
- ○ **D.** Slip the stockings over the toes before the heel.

Answers to Practice Exam II

Answers at a Glance

1. B	26. D	51. D
2. A	27. C	52. B
3. C	28. B	53. B
4. D	29. D	54. B
5. B	30. C	55. A
6. A	31. B	56. A
7. A	32. D	57. C
8. A	33. D	58. A
9. B	34. B	59. B
10. C	35. C	60. C
11. D	36. A	61. D
12. D	37. D	62. B
13. C	38. D	63. A
14. C	39. C	64. C
15. A	40. D	65. C
16. C	41. C	66. D
17. B	42. D	67. C
18. C	43. A	68. A
19. A	44. B	69. C
20. B	45. B	70. C
21. C	46. D	71. D
22. C	47. B	72. D
23. A	48. A	73. A
24. D	49. D	74. B
25. A	50. D	75. B

Rationales for Answers to Practice Exam II

1. **B.** The most accurate position to obtain a blood pressure is to have the resident in a sitting position. The blood pressure can change when the resident is lying (A and D) or standing (C).

2. **A.** The resident has a right to religious freedom, including praying when he or she feels it is necessary and in private. Asking the resident to pray silently while you perform the procedure (B), to wait until the procedure has been completed (C), or telling the resident you prayed for him or her earlier (D) does not allow the resident freedom and privacy.

3. **C.** The intake and output should be documented in the chart during each shift by the nursing assistant. Each episode is recorded on a flow sheet that is then documented in the chart. Recording the intake/output after each meal (A), every six hours (B), or every four hours (D) is incorrect because the information placed in the chart is the calculation of each shift's totals and not each occurrence of intake.

4. **D.** Hypotension is the term for low blood pressure. Tachycardia is the term for increased heart rate (A). Hypertension is the term for high blood pressure (B). Bradypnea is the term for decreased respirations (C).

5. **B.** Two hours is the maximum time before tissue damage begins. Three hours (A) is too long and increases the chances of a decubitus ulcer forming. After four hours (C), the tissue begins to break down. If the resident is left in the same position for an entire shift (D), the tissue damage would be extensive.

6. **A.** As a part of aging, our response time decreases. The inability to make decisions (B), increased agitation (C), and loss of long-term memory (D) can occur because of disease, but are not frequently caused from normal aging.

7. **A.** Shaving cream is used to soften the beard and make it easier to shave. Thoroughly drying the skin before shaving increases irritation (B). Shaving should be done following the direction of the hair, not the opposite (C). Alcohol on freshly shaved skin causes pain and drying of the skin (D).

8. **A.** The correct procedure for making sure a resident receives the correct diet is to match the resident's food tray/diet with the diet ordered usually found on the plan of care. Choice B is appropriate when the dietitian makes the resident's tray. Choice C is correct when preparing the resident to eat, and choice D is incorrect.

9. **B.** A resident's heart rate is considered within normal limits if the rate is between 60 and 100 beats per minute. A rate below 60 beats per minute is bradycardia; greater than 100 beats per minute is tachycardia, so the ranges in answers A (55–105bpm), C (45–65bpm), and D (70–120bpm) are incorrect.

10. **C.** NPO is a Latin term meaning nothing by mouth, so no tray would be delivered. Answer choices A, B, and D are all incorrect because the patient should not have anything to eat or drink when he or she is NPO. A is a liquid diet; B is a full diet, and D is part of a BRAT diet.

11. **D.** An assistive device is ordered by the physician to help with ambulation. An orthodontic device is one that is used for the teeth (A), a feeding device (B) is used for feeding, and a transfer device (C) is used for transferring the patient from a bed to a chair or elsewhere.

12. D. The right to mistreat staff and fellow residents is the only choice that is not a right of the patient. The right to privacy and dignity (A), the right of confidentiality (B), and the right to accept or refuse treatment (C) are listed in the Patient's Bill of Rights, which is a guideline for the resident's treatment, service, and expectations.

13. C. Hands that are visibly soiled should be washed with soap and water because the hand cleanser is less effective when organic material is present. The use of alcohol-based cleansers should be used after each and every contact with a resident (A). The alcohol-based cleanser is appropriate to use when soap and water are not readily available (B). After assisting a resident to the shower (D) is incorrect because the nursing assistant has been in contact with a resident and will need to use the alcohol-based cleanser or wash his or her hands.

14. C. Sensory includes hearing, seeing, touching, and speaking. The inability to read (A), ride a bike (B), or write (D) are forms of communication or mobility, not sensory.

15. A. The correct action to promote safety is to check the resident's identification before any procedure or activity. This assures the resident that you are taking steps to promote his or her safety. (B) it is disrespectful to call a resident by nicknames or first names unless the resident gives permission for you to do so. In choices (C) and (D), the CNA would not carrying out the proper safety measures and could cause harm to the resident.

16. C. Every resident has the right to his or her own religious beliefs. The nursing assistant is to respect the beliefs of the residents and not discuss or impose his or her own on the resident (A and B). The nursing assistant should not invite someone from his or her church to talk to the resident (D), unless the resident requests the visit.

17. B. Accidentally cutting a resident during grooming is considered an act of negligence because appropriate safety precautions were not taken, and the resident was injured. Physical abuse (A) is the act of purposefully causing physical injury; malpractice (C) is the wrongful act of a doctor, lawyer, or other professional that causes injury to a patient or client; and assault (D) is the crime of threat of violence to another person.

18. C. Several actions take place before a resident receives care. The nursing assistant checks the diet order against the food tray delivered. The patient must get the right food at the appropriate times. Informing the kitchen staff what type of diet the patient wants (A) or making sure the resident eats all of his or her main meal before receiving dessert (D) are not the call of the nursing assistant. Assisting the resident in washing his or her hands and face (B) can fall under the purview of the nursing assistant, but it is not the initial step before feeding a resident.

19. A. The first action is to remove the resident if he or she is in harm's way. Next, the nursing assistant should pull the alarm (B) if no one else has done so. Then, the nursing assistant should extinguish the fire if possible (C) or evacuate if instructed to do so (D).

20. B. Lying about another nursing assistant's behavior is considered defamation of character. Negligence (A) and malpractice (C) are concerned with legal responsibilities to the resident, not another nursing assistant. Insubordination (D) is a term used to describe someone who has not followed orders.

21. C. Milliliters are used to measure liquid intake and output. Ounces (A) and milligrams (B) are both solid measurements and are not used. Cups (D) is a measurement of liquid and solid, but is not used for charting intake and output.

22. **C.** The resident has a right to privacy, which includes forms of communication. Discarding any of the resident's mail, even junk mail (A), opening mail for the resident (B), or giving the mail to a family member (D) violates the resident's privacy.

23. **A.** It takes approximately 15 minutes for the mouth to regain the previous temperature after drinking or smoking. Proceeding with the temperature reading anyway (B) gives a false temperature. Waiting approximately 45 minutes (C) is not necessary. Skipping the temperature reading and taking it at the next scheduled time (D) is not following written orders as directed.

24. **D.** When an item is dropped on the floor, it has a higher probability of being contaminated and should not to be used. Picking up the linen, shaking it out, and then using it (A) or placing it on the bedside chair to use at a later time (B) might cause the resident to become sick due to the transfer of germs/bacteria. Leaving it on the floor for housekeeping to pick up (C) could cause someone to fall.

25. **A.** A Hoyer lift is a device to assist the nursing assistant with transfer of a weak or immobile resident from the bed to the chair and back again. A slide board is used to transfer the resident from the bed to a stretcher and back again (B). A brace (C) or assistive device (D) is not used in the transfer of a resident.

26. **D.** A resident files a grievance with the administration when the resident feels care or services are not what was promised. Slander is a legal term for making false statements about someone (A). Defamation refers to making a false accusation about a person's activity (B). Irritating (C) is a term used when referring to emotions.

27. **C.** Closing the curtains before beginning a procedure is an example of providing privacy. Assisting the resident onto the bedside commode and forgetting to close the curtains (A), standing beside the resident while he or she talks on the phone (B), and not providing adequate clothing while dressing the resident (D) do not properly provide the resident with his or her right to privacy.

28. **B.** Convulsions is a word used sometimes in place of seizures. Sugar in the blood (A) is sometimes used to describe diabetes. Consumption (C) is used to describe pneumonia or tuberculosis. Heart troubles (D) can be used to describe any cardiac-related conditions.

29. **D.** With a contracture, the muscle prevents the joint from moving. With arthritis (A), the joint still moves, but might be stiff and painful. A sprain (B) involves injury to the muscle or ligaments, not the bone. A fracture (C) is usually temporary and does not always involve the joint.

30. **C.** The nursing assistant does have a role in the care of a resident who is receiving intravenous therapy. The nursing assistant is responsible for monitoring the site (A), the tubing (B), checking to see that the fluid is infusing, and reporting any problems immediately (D).

31. **B.** Any problems with airway, breathing, or circulation should be reported immediately. Incontinence (A), a weak leg (C), and increased hunger (D) should be reported, but not immediately.

32. **D.** The resident has a right to refuse treatment. If the nursing assistant threatens the resident if he or she continues to refuse transfer (A), ignores the resident and transfers him or her anyway (B), or calls for help to transfer the resident because he or she might become agitated (C), the nursing assistant is not honoring the right of the resident.

33. **D.** Shortness of breath is not a sign of infection. Fever (A), swelling (B), and redness (C) are all signs of an active infection.

34. B. The first action of the CNA is to report anything out of the norm to the nurse. Choice A is an action the CNA can also do, but the first action is reporting to the nurse the change in the resident's elimination. C is not necessary, and choice D disregards the resident's concern about the change in his or her bowel habits.

35. C. Constipation is a problem that occurs with aging. The intestinal motility slows and leads to constipation. Liquid stools (A), increased stools (B), and increased appetite (D) are not due to decreased motility, but might be signs of other problems.

36. A. The only legitimate reason to restrain someone is if he or she might hurt himself or herself or someone else, and this type of restraint requires a physician's order. Using restraints as a punishment (B), to decrease the time needed to spend attending the resident (C), and to keep the resident out of the way (D) could be considered false imprisonment.

37. D. The best source is always the primary source, and from our choices the primary source would be the resident. Regarding any areas that the resident might not remember, a friend (A), family member (B), or the physician (C) may be asked.

38. D. When washing your hands, you should use a clean, dry paper towel to turn off the water to prevent contaminating areas that have been cleaned. Applying soap before wetting your hands (A) is out of order. The hands are to be wetted first; then soap is applied to one hand. Keeping hands elevated above your waist (B) and applying friction for only 5 seconds (C) would contaminate the clean areas.

39. C. For an appropriate axillary temperature to be taken, the probe needs to be placed in the center of the axilla. The arm is to be placed at the resident's side, and then the elbow bent and crossed over the chest. Placing the probe of the thermometer 1 inch under the arm (A), in the posterior 1/3 of the axilla (B), or in the anterior 1/3 of the axilla (D) are all incorrect procedures.

40. D. When obtaining a pulse rate, the rate should be counted for 60 seconds the first time it is obtained by the nursing assistant or if the pulse is irregular. Placing the fat pads of your finger over the groove in the wrist (A), using second hand or digital readout assists to keep track of the seconds (B), and lightly pressing against the radial bone (C) are proper procedures for attaining a radial pulse.

41. C. One of the important actions for every procedure is to provide privacy. Tepid water (A) chills the resident. Use of a towel to cover the resident does not supply adequate privacy (B). The feet are washed after the rest of the body (D).

42. D. Funguses like warm, moist places, so placing lotion between the toes increases the likelihood of a fungus developing. Drying the resident's hands and feet after soaking (A), reporting any breaks in the skin to the nurse (B), and soaking hands and feet at a safe temperature (C) are all parts of the procedure used for nail care.

43. A. Dentures are to be placed in an appropriately labeled container. Storing dentures on several wet paper towels (B), in a large jar filled with mouthwash (C), or in the drawer of a bedside table (D) might lead to dentures being damaged or lost.

44. B. To restore a resident to as near normal function as possible is the center of rehabilitative care. Improving the resident's capabilities (A), returning the resident to better than normal functioning (C), and preventing harm and injury (D) are goals for restorative care.

45. **B.** The resident and members of the health-care team create long-term goals for the resident. Focusing on doing things for the residents (A) and assisting the resident to remember his or her limitations (D) are negative and do not assist in improving or maintaining function. Preventing deterioration when possible (C) is a goal, but not the overall goal, of restorative care.

46. **D.** Providing privacy is a requirement for all procedures. All thermometers should be lubricated to prevent pain and injury (A). Mercury thermometers are not used any more in health-care facilities (B). The rectal temperature might be 1 degree higher (not lower) than the oral temperature (C).

47. **B.** The pulse is below normal and irregular. This pulse should be repeated before reported to the nurse. 88bpm (A), 60bpm (C), and 96bpm (D) are pulses within the normal range and have regular rhythms.

48. **A.** When a nursing assistant finds a resident down, the assistant's first action is to call for help (B) and to follow the facility's emergency plan (B). The second action is to get the AED (C) and bring it in the room; then the assistant is to check for breathing and a pulse (D).

49. **D.** The nursing assistant's responsibility includes promoting comfort and assisting the resident in the use of the bathroom, along with needs for food and fluid. Restraints are to be secured, but must have a quick release knot to remove quickly if needed, not one taped securely to remain fastened (A). Checking extremities for circulation, motion, and sensitivity over a 4-hour period (B), and documenting the reason for application of restraints in the chart (C) are the responsibility of the nurse, but the nursing assistant needs to make sure the extremity has good circulation.

50. **D.** Acknowledging the concerns of the resident and promising an appropriate action is a demonstration of good communication. The other statements, "What can I do about your life situation?" (A), "Rest awhile and you will feel better in the morning" (B), and "I can't help you right now; I am busy" (C), ignore the resident and his or her concerns.

51. **D.** If splints fit and are applied appropriately, the resident should not have pain with use; therefore, any pain should be reported immediately. Sweating (A) and difficulty in applying (C) might mean the splints need readjustment or padding. If the resident refuses to use the splint (B), the nursing assistant should report and record this as soon as possible.

52. **B.** Masks are worn for droplet or respiratory precautions. Gloves are needed for Methicillin-Resistant Staphylococcus Aureus (MRSA) precautions (A), contact precautions (C), and standard precautions (D).

53. **B.** A condom catheter is an external device and is to be removed at least once a shift for examination of the skin underneath. Do not pull the catheter onto the penis (A); the catheter is rolled on, not pulled. Too much lubrication could cause the catheter to become dislodged (C). The drainage bag should never be attached to a movable part of the bed or wheelchair (D).

54. **B.** The social worker locates resources to meet the resident's plan of care. The nurse plans the care and supervises (A). The nursing assistant is responsible to assist in carrying out the plan of care (C). The physician prescribes the resident's care (D).

55. **A.** Providing protection helps the resident not to feel embarrassed and decreases his or her anxiety. Raising the head of the bed and then rolling the resident to his or her side is an incorrect position for the head of the bed (B). Using a fracture pan (C) might cause anxiety for a larger resident and not hold contents. After use, bedpans are to be cleansed and stored in the bedside table (D).

56. B. A resident's beard is not to be trimmed unless the resident requests it. The best care of a resident with a beard is to wash (A) and comb (C) the beard at least daily and when visibly soiled (D).

57. C. Documentation of intravenous fluids is the role of the nurse. Ice cream (A), soup (B), and Jell-O (D) are fluids that should be recorded on the resident's flow sheet.

58. A. Severe cramping is not a usual response of an enema. Mild cramping might sometimes occur, but not severe cramping. Expelled brown liquid (B), increased amount of flatus (C), and large amounts of formed feces (D) are expected responses.

59. B. Securing the catheter decreases the chance of trauma to the resident if the catheter is accidently pulled. The catheter is secured in the bladder with a balloon so that it will not fall out, so answer A is not valid. Taping the catheter does not allow the resident to use the bathroom, so answer C is invalid. Securing the catheter does not actually prevent leaking, so answer D is invalid.

60. C. The licensed practical nurse carries out the medical plan under the supervision of the registered nurse. The physician prescribes the medical plan (A). The nursing assistant's role is to assist in the delivery of care (B). The physical therapist carries out orders written by the physician (D).

61. D. Spills are to be cleaned up quickly before someone is injured. Ignoring the spill (A) or attempting to delegate the spill cleanup to someone else (B and C) prolong the time the spill remains unattended.

62. B. The first step is to empty the bag and then remove it. Emptying the collection bag (C) is followed by applying skin protector around the stoma (A), and last would be reattaching the clean bag to the apparatus around the stoma (D). Gently cleanse the stoma and surrounding area. Apply a protective coating to protect the skin from being harmed by the bodily fluids.

63. A. When a resident is accidently cut while being shaved, the nursing assistant should immediately apply pressure. Applying bandages does not fall under the scope of the nursing assistant (B). Tissue paper is not appropriate and is not a sterile dressing (C). Shaving lotion has alcohol in it and will be painful if applied to a cut (D).

64. C. When a resident is depressed, he or she exhibits *decreased* interest in activities, including caring for self and eating. Loss of appetite (A), increased sleeping (B), and crying (D) are all signs of depression.

65. C. Quietly sitting with the resident as much as possible provides support, and if he or she wants to talk about fears, someone is present to listen. Ignoring the resident as much as possible (A) is unacceptable because the resident's feelings might be hurt worse if his or her feelings are not acknowledged. Telling the resident to begin to live each day to the fullest (B) and explaining to the resident that he or she might not die for awhile yet (D) can be misinterpreted as insensitive by the resident.

66. D. Oxygen is not to be removed except for a few seconds to cleanse the nose and the cannula. Removing oxygen every hour (A), every 2 hours (B), or every 8 hours (C) interrupts oxygen delivery and might jeopardize recovery for the resident.

67. C. Sitting and listening to the resident conveys caring and empathy. Changing the subject (A), introducing him or her to the other available residents on the unit (B), and telling him or her things will get better over time (D) do not respect the resident's feelings and will close off effective communication with the resident.

68. **A.** Report the incident to the resident and the nurse immediately so the resident's dentures can be replaced by the facility. Choices B and C are incorrect. The nursing assistant is being dishonest. Choice D is commendable, but it is not the nursing assistant's responsibility to replace the dentures. It is important that the nursing assistant followed all the steps in the procedure for cleaning and handling dentures.

69. **C.** Treatments are under the responsibility of the registered nurse. The nursing assistant assists in the delivering of care and reporting changes to the nurse. Discoloration is an important change that could mean the resident has decreased circulation in the extremity and should be reported immediately, not after the nursing assistant completes his or her tasks (A). Elevating the arm may not be appropriate (B), and only the nurse should remove the bandage (D).

70. **C.** Alcohol is not a stress reducer. Overindulging in food or alcohol might seem to reduce stress at the time, but in the long run the overindulgence adds to the stress. Getting plenty of rest and eating a balanced diet (A), getting involved in a new hobby (B), and exercising several times a week (D) are recommended to reduce stress.

71. **D.** Stay calm and report the behavior to the nurse caring for the resident. Any other action could escalate the anger, or you might respond in an unprofessional manner. The scene might also upset the resident.

72. **D.** It is important to the resident focus on what he or she is accomplishing with rehabilitation. The resident may need to learn new ways of caring for himself or herself, and nursing needs to assist the resident as needed, but not do everything for him or her (A). The nursing assistant should listen to the resident and show empathy not sympathy (B). Allow the resident to talk about losses, but help him or her to focus on goals for the future (C).

73. **A.** Slander is making a false accusation about someone that injures his or her character or reputation. Malpractice (B) is the break in a standard of care or standard of practice by a member of a profession. Negligence (C) is the failing of someone to act or acting in a way that injures someone. Assault (D) is threatening to harm someone or leading someone to believe you will harm him or her.

74. **B.** Sitting and listening to the resident conveys caring and empathy. Calling the family may not respect the resident's feelings and may close off effective communication with the resident (C). Giving the resident sleeping medication would be the wrong use of a medication and delays the healing process (A), and calling the doctor is not in the scope of the nursing assistant(D).

75. **B.** Elastic stockings need to be wrinkle free to prevent discomfort and to minimize the possibility of pressure ulcers from the wrinkles. Pulling the stocking up smoothly over the legs (A), supporting the resident's foot at the heel (C), and slipping the stockings over the toes before the heel (D) are all correct actions, but are not critical steps.

Practice Exam III

This exam consists of 75 questions that reflect the material covered in this book. The questions are representative of the types of questions you should expect to see on the Certified Nursing Assistant Examination; however, they are not intended to match exactly what is on the exam.

Some of the questions require that you deduce the best possible answer. Often, you are asked to identify the best course of action to take in a given situation. Read the questions carefully and thoroughly before you attempt to answer them. For best results, treat this exam as if it were the actual examination. When you take it, time yourself, read carefully, and answer all the questions to the best of your ability.

The answers to all the questions appear in "Answers to Practice Exam III." Check your letter answers against those in the answer key, and then read the explanations provided. You might also want to return to the appropriate chapters in the book to review the material associated with any questions you have answered incorrectly. Also, review the tables in Appendix A, "Nursing Assistant Test Cross-Reference," which maps the questions in the nine categories of questions that you will see on the written exam, as listed by the National Nurse Aide Assessment Program:

► Member of health-care team

► Activities of daily living

► Client rights

► Basic nursing skills

► Emotional and mental health needs

► Communication

► Restorative skills

► Spiritual and cultural issues

► Legal and ethical behavior

Exam Questions

1. The CNA who willfully does not provide care to a resident is guilty of which of the following?

   ○ **A.** Negligence

   ○ **B.** Malpractice

   ○ **C.** Slander

   ○ **D.** Assault

2. Which of the following is a description of a stage one decubitus ulcer?

   ○ **A.** Redness that does not turn white when pressed

   ○ **B.** Open area with redness

   ○ **C.** Black area

   ○ **D.** Open area with visible bone

3. A nursing assistant is offered a $10 tip by a family member of a resident for taking good care of the member's mother. Which of the following is the best course of action for the nursing assistant?

   ○ **A.** Ask another nursing assistant what he or she would do.

   ○ **B.** Say thank you and take the money.

   ○ **C.** Refuse to accept the money.

   ○ **D.** Instruct the family member to give the money to the supervisor.

4. Which of the following is not part of the procedure when documenting in the medical record?

   ○ **A.** Writing in pencil

   ○ **B.** Writing in pen

   ○ **C.** Crossing through mistakes and initialing them

   ○ **D.** Using correct spelling

5. Which of the following behaviors is considered a demonstration of caring?

   ○ **A.** The timely completion of an assignment

   ○ **B.** Taking the time to listen to the resident

   ○ **C.** Obtaining the vital signs for the unit before lunch

   ○ **D.** Not changing the resident when he or she is soiled

6. The nursing assistant is ready to enter Mrs. Jane Smith's room to care for her. Which of the following is the best way to approach Mrs. Smith?

   ○ **A.** "Hi, I am assigned to care for you today."

   ○ **B.** "Hi, Jane, I am Sue, your nursing assistant."

   ○ **C.** "Good morning, Mrs. Smith. I am Mrs. Jones, the nursing assistant on duty today. How may I help you?"

   ○ **D.** "Time to wake up and get moving, Mrs. Smith. I have a lot to accomplish today."

7. When a resident refuses a bath, the nursing assistant should perform which of the following actions?

   ○ **A.** Inform the resident that everyone must take a bath when it is scheduled.

   ○ **B.** The charge nurse does not need to be informed that resident did not take a bath.

   ○ **C.** Go ahead and bathe the resident.

   ○ **D.** Respect the resident's wishes.

8. When residents have visitors, it is important for the nursing assistant to do which of the following?

   ○ **A.** Provide snacks for the resident and family members.

   ○ **B.** Provide privacy.

   ○ **C.** Remain close enough to hear the resident's conversation.

   ○ **D.** Leave the intercom on in case the resident needs assistance.

9. Which of the following is not included in the resident's right to information?

   ○ **A.** Latest hospital inspection results

   ○ **B.** Notification in advance of a change of room or roommate

   ○ **C.** Right to file a complaint with the state survey agency

   ○ **D.** Right to free or reduced medical care

10. Which of the following best defines quadriplegia?

   ○ **A.** Flaccid lower extremities

   ○ **B.** No movement in all four extremities

   ○ **C.** Inability to move the left side

   ○ **D.** No feeling in both feet

11. When the nursing assistant is communicating with a resident who is suffering from memory loss, which of the following constitutes appropriate communication skills?

    ○ **A.** Sitting beside the resident and listening to him or her.

    ○ **B.** Ignoring the resident and continuing to work.

    ○ **C.** Laughing at what the resident is saying.

    ○ **D.** Asking the resident not to talk nonsense.

12. Which of the following creates an environment for effective communication with a resident who is visually impaired?

    ○ **A.** Making sure the light in the room is not too bright

    ○ **B.** Placing rugs on the floor so the resident is not too shocked by the cold floor

    ○ **C.** Making sure the resident's glasses and other visual aids are within reach

    ○ **D.** Turning up the volume on the television so the resident can hear because he or she has trouble seeing

13. What is the appropriate action of the nursing assistant when the resident asks for time alone with her husband?

    ○ **A.** Leave the room, but keep the door open.

    ○ **B.** Provide privacy for the resident.

    ○ **C.** Tell the resident that it is best if the husband comes back at a later time.

    ○ **D.** Call the physician and clarify the resident's physical condition.

14. Which of the following substances should be used to cleanse the drain on the urinary drainage bag after emptying it?

    ○ **A.** Alcohol

    ○ **B.** Soap and water

    ○ **C.** Nothing, just allow the drain to air dry

    ○ **D.** Peroxide

15. Which of the following actions is a violation of the resident's right to privacy and security?

    ○ **A.** Removing the resident's clothes from his or her room without permission

    ○ **B.** Asking the resident's permission to give the resident a bath

    ○ **C.** Gently waking the resident for breakfast

    ○ **D.** Offering the resident the opportunity to wash his or her face and brush his or her teeth before serving breakfast.

16. Which of the following best defines an ombudsman?

   ○ **A.** A person who represents a resident and investigates his or her complaint

   ○ **B.** A nurse representative who assures quality care

   ○ **C.** A person appointed by the court to handle an estate

   ○ **D.** A union representative

17. Which of the following is a sign that a resident is being physically or verbally abused?

   ○ **A.** A daughter discusses changes in care with her mother.

   ○ **B.** The resident's sleeping medication is withheld because the resident would not take a bath.

   ○ **C.** A son does not return his father for several hours whenever they go out to lunch.

   ○ **D.** The wrong medication is given to a resident.

18. Which of the following is an example of maintaining client confidentiality?

   ○ **A.** The CNA goes around the unit asking family and residents about their personal lives.

   ○ **B.** The CNA reports information to the CNA who is assigned to take care of the resident on the incoming shift.

   ○ **C.** The dietary aide brings the resident's chart to the room and leaves it for visitors to read.

   ○ **D.** The CNA shares the resident's HIV status with new employees.

19. While the CNA was assisting a new resident with his morning care, the CNA noticed that the new resident had several bruises in various stages of healing. The correct action of the CNA is to:

   ○ **A.** Question the resident about the bruises.

   ○ **B.** Report to the bruises to the nurse.

   ○ **C.** Make a note in the chart.

   ○ **D.** Call the family and demand to know what caused the bruising.

20. The CNA is asked to take the temperature of a resident who has been vomiting. Which of the routes is most appropriate?

   ○ **A.** Rectal

   ○ **B.** Axillary

   ○ **C.** Tympanic

   ○ **D.** Oral

21. Which position is correct for the CNA who is assisting a resident from a chair to the bed?

    ○ **A.** Standing to the side of the resident, placing the hands under the resident's armpits, and lifting

    ○ **B.** Moving the resident to the edge of the chair; then, standing with feet apart, bending the knees and placing the arms under the resident's arms and lifting

    ○ **C.** Moving the resident to the edge of the chair; then, standing with feet apart, bending the knees, placing the forearms under the resident's arms and lifting

    ○ **D.** Facing the resident, feet apart, apply the gait belt to the resident, and lifting the resident via the gait belt.

22. What is the best position for the CNA to use in order to prevent injury to his or her back or neck while bathing a resident?

    ○ **A.** Move as close to the resident as possible.

    ○ **B.** Work from the foot of the bed.

    ○ **C.** Raise the bed to a comfortable level.

    ○ **D.** Stand on the resident's weak side.

23. Which of the following procedures requires the CNA to wear gloves in order to adhere to standard precautions?

    ○ **A.** Setting up the dinner tray

    ○ **B.** Taking out the trash

    ○ **C.** Providing oral care

    ○ **D.** Providing hair care

24. The best position for a resident who is unconscious and needs oral care is which of the following?

    ○ **A.** High-Fowlers

    ○ **B.** Side-lying

    ○ **C.** Trendelenburg

    ○ **D.** Supine

25. What is the most important action the CNA can perform to prevent the spread of infections?

    ○ **A.** Wearing gloves

    ○ **B.** Adhering to precautions

    ○ **C.** Encouraging residents to bathe everyday

    ○ **D.** Hand washing

26. Which is part of the dress code for CNAs working in long-term care facilities?

   ○ **A.** T-shirt, clean shoes, and tight fitting pants

   ○ **B.** Clean and tidy uniform scrubs, color specified by the facility

   ○ **C.** Loose pants and tight shirts to prevent the possibility of getting dirty

   ○ **D.** Jeans, uniform top, and lab coat

27. What action by the CNA is acceptable when a resident has his or her room door open?

   ○ **A.** Knock before entering.

   ○ **B.** Walk in and ask the resident if he or she meant to leave it open.

   ○ **C.** Ask the nurse to tell the resident to close the door.

   ○ **D.** Wait till the patient exits the room before going in.

28. Which of the following selections could be grounds for legal action by a resident?

   ○ **A.** Assisting the patient with a bath at his or her request

   ○ **B.** Taking the resident for a walk outside when the family asked the CNA to keep the resident inside

   ○ **C.** Making unwelcomed explicit or implied sexual statements to the resident

   ○ **D.** Mistakenly feeding the resident culturally taboo foods

29. When a sharps container is full it should be

   ○ **A.** Shaken to be sure it is full

   ○ **B.** Taken off the wall, closed, and set in the dirty utility room

   ○ **C.** Closed, sealed, and disposed of according to facility safety policy

   ○ **D.** Emptied into a larger container for disposal

30. When asked by the nurse to be in the room for a sterile procedure, the CNA knows that the main goal implied by the term "sterile" is to keep the area free of pathogens by

   ○ **A.** Avoiding touching equipment or other objects placed in the sterile field

   ○ **B.** Setting up the sterile field

   ○ **C.** Positioning and prepping the resident for the procedure

   ○ **D.** Guarding the sterile field once it is set up

31. What is the best response of the CNA when a resident requests that his or her toenails be trimmed?

   ○ **A.** The CNA cleans and trims the toenails.

   ○ **B.** The CNA notifies the nurse of the resident's request so the nurse can contact the podiatrist.

   ○ **C.** The CNA informs the nurse that it is time for him to cut his toenails.

   ○ **D.** The CNA provides the resident with nail clippers.

32. What should the nursing assistant do when he or she discovers a resident has edema?

   ○ **A.** Carefully clean the area.

   ○ **B.** Place compression stockings on the resident.

   ○ **C.** Notify the nurse.

   ○ **D.** Do nothing.

33. What is the best way to encourage social interaction?

   ○ **A.** Speak to all residents, even when they cannot take part in the conversation.

   ○ **B.** Sit annoying residents away from other residents.

   ○ **C.** Do not talk to residents who speak a different language.

   ○ **D.** Speak loudly to all residents.

34. Which of the following signs does not indicate the patient may be in pain?

   ○ **A.** Facial grimacing

   ○ **B.** Smiling

   ○ **C.** Holding an area

   ○ **D.** Crying

35. What is the final action the CNA should take when performing toileting?

   ○ **A.** Walk the resident to the bathroom.

   ○ **B.** Wash his or her hands.

   ○ **C.** Flush the toilet.

   ○ **D.** Clean the bathroom area.

36. A CNA is reviewing a patient's diet during shift change. Which of the following actions would be indicated for a resident who has difficulty sleeping?

    ○ **A.** Allow the resident to drink fluids until he or she is ready to go to bed.

    ○ **B.** Offer tea and coffee after 6 p.m.

    ○ **C.** Encourage residents to drink only caffeine-free beverages later in the day.

    ○ **D.** Offer sodas with dinner.

37. There are times when the blood pressure cannot be taken in one arm. Which of the following sites is recommended to take a blood pressure?

    ○ **A.** An arm that is paralyzed

    ○ **B.** An arm on the side where the resident has had a mastectomy

    ○ **C.** An arm without any abnormalities

    ○ **D.** An arm with an IV infusing

38. A resident tells the nursing assistant that her arm is uncomfortable at the place she has an IV. The nursing assistant knows to report which of following signs to the nurse?

    ○ **A.** Skin pink and warm around the site

    ○ **B.** Swollen and red skin around the site

    ○ **C.** Dressing dry around the site

    ○ **D.** Clear, clean IV insertion site

39. A nursing assistant has just suffered a needle stick while working with a resident who is positive for AIDS. Which of the following is the most important action the nursing assist should take?

    ○ **A.** Wash the site.

    ○ **B.** Notify the nurse.

    ○ **C.** Tell the resident.

    ○ **D.** Call the doctor.

40. What does having a paralyzed side mean?

    ○ **A.** The arm and leg on one side of the body is weak.

    ○ **B.** The arm on one side is malformed.

    ○ **C.** The face is saggy.

    ○ **D.** The arm and leg on one side of the body is flaccid.

41. Which of the following is the most appropriate skin care for a resident who is on nasal oxygen?

   ○ **A.** Place Vaseline around the nostrils.

   ○ **B.** Clean the nostrils with soap and water every two hours.

   ○ **C.** Make sure to check the pressure areas and reposition tubing every two hours.

   ○ **D.** Use petroleum jelly a couple of times a day.

42. To obtain the most accurate patient weight, the nursing assistant should weigh the resident when?

   ○ **A.** First thing in the morning

   ○ **B.** Later in the afternoon

   ○ **C.** Before he or she goes to the bathroom

   ○ **D.** After exercise

43. When correcting a mistake in the chart, the nursing assistant knows it is best to do which of the following?

   ○ **A.** Scribble out any mistakes.

   ○ **B.** If a mistake is made, the CNA is to cross out the mistake by putting one line through it and initialing it.

   ○ **C.** CNAs do not write in a resident's chart.

   ○ **D.** Use white out when a small mistake is made.

44. Which of the following is *not* a sign that an elderly resident may be suffering from a urinary tract infection?

   ○ **A.** Confusion

   ○ **B.** Increased urge to urine

   ○ **C.** Burning sensation with urination

   ○ **D.** Increased thirst

45. A resident who sometimes has episodes of aggressive behavior is admitted to the Alzheimer's unit. Which response by the CNA is important for safety when the resident is aggressive?

   ○ **A.** Tell the resident that if his or her behavior does not change, you will have the nurse put him or her in restraints.

   ○ **B.** Talk loudly and use force if necessary to subdue the resident, and then tell the nurse.

   ○ **C.** Speak quietly and leave the situation if you can, and tell the nurse before returning to the resident.

   ○ **D.** Tell the resident that you do not have time for this behavior and to calm down.

46. The CNA is responsible to do which of following when providing post-mortem care?

○ **A.** Remove all the tubes.

○ **B.** Remove the dentures.

○ **C.** Clean the body for viewing by the family members.

○ **D.** Remove dressings.

47. Select all the steps below that are *not* part of obtaining an oral temperature using an electronic thermometer (not all the steps are listed).

○ **A.** Wash hands.

○ **B.** Offer the resident some fluids before taking temperature.

○ **C.** Place probe on the thermometer.

○ **D.** Record temperature and mode used to access according to agency policy.

48. A resident with a stroke is fitted for a leg brace. Which intervention is *most important* when caring for this resident?

○ **A.** Skin care

○ **B.** Elimination assistance

○ **C.** Increased fluids

○ **D.** Increased ambulation

49. The most accurate reading for a radial pulse will be to count it for a full

○ **A.** 15 seconds and multiply by 4

○ **B.** 60 seconds

○ **C.** 30 seconds and multiply by 2

○ **D.** 10 seconds and multiply by 6

50. For an accurate blood pressure reading

○ **A.** The arm the blood pressure reading is being taken from should be at heart level.

○ **B.** The resident should sit comfortably with legs crossed.

○ **C.** The resident does not need to avoid talking while taking the CNA obtains his or her blood pressure.

○ **D.** The resident can drink while the CNA obtains his or her blood pressure.

51. When the nursing assistant cleanses the genital and rectal areas, he or she is performing which of the following?

  ○ **A.** P.M. care

  ○ **B.** A.M. care

  ○ **C.** Perineal care

  ○ **D.** Hygiene care

52. Which of the following is a measure to prevent falls?

  ○ **A.** Put all side rails up after the resident is in bed.

  ○ **B.** Remove the bedside table from close to the bed.

  ○ **C.** Put on the bed alarm before leaving the room.

  ○ **D.** Turn all the lights off and close the door to the resident's room.

53. When the doctor asks you to get the nurse "stat," when does he mean for you to do it?

  ○ **A.** In 5 minutes or so

  ○ **B.** When you finish what you are doing

  ○ **C.** Before he leaves

  ○ **D.** Instantly

54. When is an ostomy pouch emptied?

  ○ **A.** When the pouch is full

  ○ **B.** Every two hours

  ○ **C.** Every day with a.m. care

  ○ **D.** Every shift

55. When the CNA notices that he or she is becoming impatient with a resident, he or she should do which of the following?

  ○ **A.** He or she should leave the room (if able) and come back when feeling less impatient.

  ○ **B.** The CNA should tell the resident that he or she is beginning to irritate him or her.

  ○ **C.** The CNA should speak with the nurse about his or her feelings.

  ○ **D.** The CNA should tell the family members that his or her loved one is irritating.

56. When the resident asks to see a pastor of his or her faith, the CNA knows to

  ○ **A.** Call a local church to have someone come visit the resident.

  ○ **B.** Tell the nurse that the resident has requested to talk to a pastor.

  ○ **C.** Call the doctor and see if the resident is allowed to have outside visitors.

  ○ **D.** Tell the resident that you are a minister at your church and that you can help them.

57. When the CNA is helping a resident perform passive range-of-motion movements, the most effective indicator that movement should be stopped occurs when the resident reports

   ○ **A.** Stiffness

   ○ **B.** Weakness

   ○ **C.** Pain

   ○ **D.** Muscle size increasing

58. A precaution against what type of danger requires the nursing assistant to wear a mask?

   ○ **A.** Blood borne

   ○ **B.** Standard

   ○ **C.** Contact

   ○ **D.** Droplet

59. Which of the following medical terms is used for describing a broken bone?

   ○ **A.** Fracture

   ○ **B.** Sprain

   ○ **C.** Strain

   ○ **D.** Laceration

60. When assisting the resident to ambulate using a gait-transfer belt, the resident should be asked if

   ○ **A.** He or she would like the CNA to stand in front of or behind him or her.

   ○ **B.** He or she feels steady, or if he or she has any nausea or dizziness.

   ○ **C.** He or she would like to wear headphones.

   ○ **D.** The CNA can bring his or her cell phone to answer emails while assisting the resident.

61. The number one way to prevent contamination from resident to resident is for the CNA to

   ○ **A.** Close the resident's door.

   ○ **B.** Wash his or her hands.

   ○ **C.** Bathe the resident every day.

   ○ **D.** Clean the resident's bathroom after use by visitors.

62. Which of the following behaviors is considered a violation of the resident's right to privacy?

   ○ **A.** The nurse telling the provider that the resident is not eating

   ○ **B.** A family member telling the nurse that it is the resident's birthday

   ○ **C.** The CNA telling a visitor from church that the resident refuses to take his or her medications

   ○ **D.** The doctor telling the CNA caring for the resident that he or she may be experiencing pain when moved

63. What is the first action of the CNA when he or she notices a reddened area on the right hip when turning the resident in bed?

   ○ **A.** Gently massage the area.

   ○ **B.** Tell the nurse.

   ○ **C.** Apply lotion to the skin.

   ○ **D.** Turn the resident more often.

64. The wife asks to pray with the resident before leaving, but visiting hours are over. Which of the following is the CNA's best response?

   ○ **A.** To tell the wife that you are sorry, but visiting hours are over. Please come back tomorrow.

   ○ **B.** To pray with the wife and the resident.

   ○ **C.** To provide the wife and the resident privacy to pray.

   ○ **D.** To let the wife know that the chapel is provided for praying.

65. A Jewish resident asks the CNA if he is getting kosher meals. The CNA realizes that kosher meals are

   ○ **A.** Meals that are specially prepared when requested by Jewish residents who adhere to the Jewish culture

   ○ **B.** Religious meals made for special days in the Jewish culture

   ○ **C.** Prepared in the same way as regular meals.

   ○ **D.** Prepared by rabbis and delivered by family members

66. Which of the following is the best position in which to place the resident to assist with oral care?

   ○ **A.** Left lateral

   ○ **B.** High Fowler's

   ○ **C.** Supine

   ○ **D.** Lithotomy

67. The safest way to dress a resident who has a problem with weakness on one side of the body is to begin with the

   ○ **A.** Unaffected side

   ○ **B.** Strong side

   ○ **C.** Weak side

   ○ **D.** Feet first

68. Which of the following are behaviors commonly related to a resident with mild cognitive impairment (dementia)?

    ○ **A.** Memory problems

    ○ **B.** Inability to dress

    ○ **C.** Inability to feed self

    ○ **D.** Unable to ambulate

69. Which of the following actions will help to prevent injury to the skin from a cold compress?

    ○ **A.** Do not remove the compress until it has reached room temperature.

    ○ **B.** Place a washcloth between the cold pack and the skin.

    ○ **C.** Place a heating pad on the skin after the cold pack is removed.

    ○ **D.** Wash the area after removing the cold pack.

70. The resident who has had a stroke may have difficulties swallowing and be placed on aspiration precautions. Which of the following actions are important for the CNA to take to prevent aspiration?

    ○ **A.** Provide only liquids to the resident.

    ○ **B.** Allow the resident to sit in any position to eat.

    ○ **C.** Feed the resident small amounts of food.

    ○ **D.** Wait to provide oral care until bedtime.

71. What team member is responsible for developing a discharge plan for a resident?

    ○ **A.** Social worker

    ○ **B.** Dietitian

    ○ **C.** CNA

    ○ **D.** Physical therapist

72. Which of the following is an example of an assistive device?

    ○ **A.** Cane

    ○ **B.** Walker

    ○ **C.** Wheelchair

    ○ **D.** All of the above

73. Of the following selections, which one, when performed by the CNA, will most assist the resident to reach his or her highest possible functional and physical status?

- ○ **A.** Help the resident with activities when he or she becomes frustrated.
- ○ **B.** Wait to give the resident praise until he or she shows great improvements in functional ability.
- ○ **C.** Promote independence with activities of daily living.
- ○ **D.** Allow the resident to work on his or plan of care when he or she becomes fatigued.

74. Select all that apply to the goals of restorative care.

- ○ **A.** Decrease falls and injuries.
- ○ **B.** Promote activity.
- ○ **C.** Promote mobility.
- ○ **D.** Increase muscle strength.

75. New residents may grieve the loss of their independence. Which of the following will aid the new resident in the adjustment?

- ○ **A.** Making all the resident's choices for him or her
- ○ **B.** Keeping the resident separated from other residents until he or she becomes comfortable
- ○ **C.** Making sure to remove any personal items that might remind him or her of home
- ○ **D.** Encouraging the resident to participate in his or her favorite activities.

Answers to Practice Exam III

Answers at a Glance

1. A	26. B	51. C
2. A	27. A	52. C
3. C	28. C	53. D
4. A	29. C	54. D
5. B	30. A	55. A
6. C	31. B	56. B
7. D	32. C	57. C
8. B	33. A	58. D
9. D	34. B	59. A
10. B	35. B	60. B
11. A	36. C	61. B
12. C	37. C	62. C
13. B	38. B	63. B
14. A	39. A	64. C
15. A	40. D	65. A
16. A	41. C	66. B
17. B	42. A	67. C
18. B	43. B	68. A
19. B	44. D	69. B
20. D	45. C	70. C
21. D	46. C	71. A
22. C	47. B	72. D
23. C	48. A	73. C
24. B	49. B	74. A, B, C, D
25. D	50. A	75. D

Rationales for Answers to Practice Exam III

1. **A.** The CNA is licensed and has the potential to be charged with negligence for not providing care to a resident. Malpractice (B), slander (C), and assault (D) are legal terms that do not apply to this situation.

2. **A.** Stage one of a pressure sore is redness. Open area with redness is indicative of stage two (B). Black area is indicative of stage three (C), and open area with visible bone is indicative of stage four (D).

3. **C.** It is unethical to accept money from a resident when employed to take care of that person. Facilities have policies regarding gifts and tips, so answer A is incorrect. Choices B and D are forms of accepting money, which make them incorrect.

4. **A.** The chart is a legal document. Entries into the chart are written with pen (B) and are not erased. If a factual or typographical error is made (D), a single line is made through the error, and then it is initialed (C).

5. **B.** Listening to the resident when he or she is talking demonstrates caring, showing value to the resident as a person. Timely completion of an assignment (A) and obtaining vital signs for the unit before lunch (C) are tasks and are not forms of caring. Not changing the resident when soiled (D) is considered neglect.

6. **C.** A professional should introduce himself or herself by surname and title and show respect to the resident by referring to the resident by his or her surname. The options in answers A, B, and D are incorrect because they either do not show respect to the resident or are not professional.

7. **D.** The resident has the right to refuse care. The nurse does not need to be informed of the refusal is incorrect. The nurse should be informed of the resident's refusal, but this can be done as soon as the nursing assistant is able (B). Informing the resident that everyone must take a bath when it is scheduled (A) or simply proceeding to bathe the resident anyway (C) does not respect the rights of the resident.

8. **B.** Residents have the right to privacy at all times, including when family is visiting. Providing snacks for the resident and family members (A), although hospitable, is not a responsibility of the nursing assistant. Remaining close enough to hear the conversation (C) and leaving the intercom on (D) do not provide privacy.

9. **D.** Nursing home residents have the right to know the costs for services rendered, but not to demand free or reduced medical care. (A) Residents have the right to information, including the regulations of the home. (B) The resident has the right to participate in decisions about his or her roommate, and he or she also has (C) the right to file complaints and grievances without fear of reprisal.

10. **B.** Quadriplegia is the result of all four limbs being paralyzed. Flaccid lower extremities (A) refers to both lower extremities being paralyzed. Inability to move the left side (C) refers to someone who is hemiplegic. The loss of feeling in both feet (D) is numbness, not paralysis.

11. **A.** The nursing assistant demonstrates caring by sitting and listening to the resident. Ignoring (B), laughing (C), or demanding (D) the resident stop talking is inappropriate and demonstrates a lack of care for the resident and her condition.

12. **C.** Visual aids need to be within reach of the resident in order for the resident to be able to use them when needed. Making sure the light in the room is not too bright (A) is wrong because the light might need to be brighter for someone who is visually impaired. Placing rugs on the floor so the resident will not be too shocked by the cold floor (B) is wrong because a visually impaired resident can easily trip and fall on loose rugs. Turning up the volume on the television so the resident can hear because he or she has trouble seeing (D) is wrong because the other senses might heighten, not lessen.

13. **B.** The facility should provide the resident privacy for sexual expression. Many residents in long-term care facilities have an active sex life. Leaving the door open (A) or telling the resident to ask the husband to come at a later time (C) is a violation of the resident's rights. Calling the physician is not included under the nursing assistant's scope of practice (D).

14. **A.** The first step in emptying the urinary drainage bag is to release the clamp and allow the urine to flow into a graduate. Then reclamp the tubing and cleanse the end with alcohol. (B) Soap and water, (C) air-drying, and (D) peroxide do not cleanse the tip of tubing appropriately to prevent infection.

15. **A.** Removing any items might be considered a violation of the resident's rights. Asking the resident's permission to give him or her a bath (B), gently waking the resident for breakfast (C), and offering to wash his or her face and brush his or her teeth before serving breakfast (D) show respect for the resident and his or her rights.

16. **A.** An ombudsman is the person who represents a resident and investigates complaints. A nurse representative who assures quality care (B) is the quality care manager. A person appointed by the court to handle an estate (C) is a guardian. A union representative (D) helps the employees, not the residents.

17. **B.** Withholding medication as a form of punishment is considered abuse. A daughter discussing changes in care with her mother (A) or a son who does not return his father for several hours whenever they go out to lunch (C) is not demonstrating physical or verbal abuse. Giving the wrong medication to a resident (D) is an example of malpractice if the resident is harmed by the error.

18. **B.** The resident has the right to confidentiality. Unless the CNA is assigned to the care of the resident, the CNA should not seek (A) or share (D) information about the resident. All persons who are using the chart must protect the information properly and place the chart in a secure area after using it (C).

19. **B.** All health-care persons have a moral and legal responsibility to report suspected elder abuse to the authorities. A and C—assessing the bruises and inquiring—are documented by the nurse (D). The CNA should not be confrontational with the family or the resident.

20. **D.** Rectal temperatures reflect closely the body's core temperature (A). B and C may not provide an accurate temperature.

21. **D.** This choice lists all the correct steps to prevent injury to the CNA and the resident in a transfer from a chair. Choices A, B, and C may put the CNA and/or the resident at risk for harm.

22. **C.** Adjusting the bed to an appropriate height prevents having to bend the back while bathing the resident. Positions A, B, and D will not prevent bending, reaching, and twisting the body, and all may lead to back injury.

23. **C.** When the CNA provides oral care, he or she is likely to come in contact with body fluids. The care detailed in answers A, B, and C does not put the CNA at risk for exposure to body fluids.

24. **B.** The side-lying position is the position of choice to help the fluids to flow out of the mouth to prevent aspiration. All other positions are inappropriate for an unconscious patient.

25. **D.** Handwashing is the most important action to prevent infections. A and B are correct actions, but not the most important. Answer C does not prevent infection, and if the resident's skin becomes too dry, the skin can crack and provide an entry for infections.

26. **B.** Facilities designate a particular dress code that includes a particular color of loose-fitting scrubs that are clean and neat. T-shirts (A), jeans (C), or tight shirts (C) are generally not a part of the CNA's dress code for duty.

27. **A.** Every member of the health-care team should treat the residents with respect and knock every time before entering a room. Even if the door is standing wide open, knock and wait to be bade entrance before going into a resident's room. That room is his or her personal space. Options B, C, and D do not demonstrate respect of the resident's private space.

28. **C.** Sexual harassment or making unwelcome sexually explicit or implied statements to residents is abusive and can be grounds for resident grievance or legal action. Option A, helping a resident at his or her request, is part of the CNA's responsibility. Options B and D are wrong, but are not grounds for legal actions.

29. **C.** When a sharps container is full, the container should be closed, sealed, and disposed of according to the facility's safety policy. The actions of A, B, and D increase the chance of someone being exposed to contaminated sharps.

30. **A.** When the CNA assists with sterile procedures (catheter insertions, applying a dressing), the CNA is to avoid touching equipment or other objects in the sterile field. B, C, and D are the responsibility of the nurse.

31. **B.** Only a podiatrist should trim the toenails of geriatric patients because older persons have decreased circulation and small cuts could become infected.

32. **C.** When a change is noticed in the resident, it needs to be reported to the nurse as soon as possible. Choices A and D can be done, but reporting a change to the nurse is the most important response of the CNA. Choice B is incorrect because a doctor is to prescribe compression stocking.

33. **A.** Residents need social interaction for psychological health. The best way to encourage social interaction is speak to all residents even when they are unable to be a part of the interaction. Choices B, C, and D are actions that do not encourage socialization.

34. **B.** The CNA should observe the resident's body language for signs of pain. If the resident is smiling, he or she is probably not in pain. Choices A, C, and D are nonverbal indications that the resident may be in pain.

35. **B.** When the CNA is assisting the resident with toileting, it is important for the CNA to wash his or her hands. Choices A, C, and D are steps in assisting the resident, but not the final step.

36. **C.** Caffeinated beverages should be limited to earlier in the day and restricted closer to bedtime to promote sleep.

37. **C.** Due to the possibility of a false reading or injuring the arm, a resident's blood pressure should be taken in an arm that does not have an IV (D), that is not on the side of a mastectomy (B), or that is not paralyzed (A).

38. B. The sign of an infiltrated IV site is a swollen, red, painful area that may ooze fluid from the insertion site. Choices A, C, and D are signs of a healthy skin and IV site.

39. A. The needle stick site needs to be washed thoroughly immediately, and then the incident should be reported to the nurse in order to follow facility protocol for needle sticks (B). Choices C and D are the responsibility of the nurse on duty.

40. D. When a resident's chart states that he or she has a paralyzed side, it means that his or her arm and leg on one side of the body is flaccid. A stroke or spinal cord injury can cause paralysis of the body below the injury site.

41. C. When a resident is using an oxygen device, the CNA should check the skin around the device frequently for any skin breakdown, and then reposition the device. Many oxygen delivery methods use tubing or edges that put pressure on the nares, top of the nose, cheeks, or ears when in use.

42. A. First thing in the morning is the time of day to acquire the most accurate weight. The actions in B, C, and D change the weight with the activity.

43. B. The proper procedure when a charting mistake occurs is to put one line through the mistake and initial it. Choices A, C, and D are actions that appear something is being covered up instead of corrected.

44. D. Increased thirst is a sign of increase sugar levels or dehydration, not a UTI. A sign that an elderly resident may have a urinary tract infection include all options A, B, and C.

45. C. To diffuse aggressive behavior, the CNA should leave the situation if he or she can and return later. Option A is considered threatening to the resident and may be considered assault. Option B is opposite of what is needed to calm the resident. The best course is to have a calm demeanor and be understanding. Option D would escalate an aggressive resident.

46. C. If time permits, the CNA is responsible to clean the body, comb the hair, and remove visible blood or other body fluids before the family visits. Option A and D are incorrect because the CNA does not remove any tubes or dressings connected to the body. Option B—the dentures are to be cleaned, placed in the mouth, and sent to the funeral home with the resident.

47. B. A, C, and D are steps for obtaining an oral temperature using an electronic thermometer. The steps are as follows:

a. Wash hands.

b. Remove the thermometer from the charger.

c. Place probe on the thermometer.

d. Gently place in resident's mouth under the side of the tongue at the back of the mouth.

e. Ask resident to close mouth around probe with lips closed.

f. Remove probe when beep sounds and see temperature display on the thermometer.

g. Eject probe into proper receptacle.

h. Clean thermometer and replace on charger.

i. Record temperature and mode used to access according to agency policy.

Option B is incorrect because offering fluids would cause a false reading for an oral temperature. If resident has just finished having a drink, then the CNA should wait 15 minutes before taking the oral temperature.

48. A. A resident with a new leg brace will need frequent skin care. The brace will need to be examined to ensure that the edges are not putting pressure on the skin that may lead to skin breakdown and skin ulcers. Options B, C, and D are essential for most residents.

49. B. A radial pulse is taken for a full 60 seconds, and the number is recorded on the resident's chart. Many residents have irregular, fast, or slow heartbeats, and to obtain an accurate reading, the pulse should be counted for a full 60 seconds; the number is recorded on the resident's chart. Options A, C, and D have been used, but they are not best practices.

50. A. Research findings support option A, the arm at heart level, and further states that feet should be uncrossed (B) and flat on the floor, and no talking (C) or drinking (D) while the blood pressure is being taken for the most accurate reading.

51. C. Perineal care is the cleansing of the genital and rectal areas. Option A is night time facial and tooth cleansing. Option B is morning time facial cleansing and tooth brushing. Option D is not a term that is used in care.

52. C. Bed alarms are to alert the staff to the resident's getting out of bed so that the staff can respond to assist as needed. Options A, B, and C are incorrect and increase chances of the resident's falling (A). When side rails are elevated, the resident may attempt to climb out of bed (B). The bedside table should be close to the resident in case he or she is looking for an item on the table when he or she wakes up, and (D) having all the lights off may cause the resident to become disoriented.

53. D. The term STAT means to accomplish the task immediately. Options A, B, and C do not reflect the definition for STAT.

54. D. An ostomy pouch should be changed every shift so that the amount of output for the shift can be added to the 24-hour Intake and Output record. Options A, B, and C are incorrect and may cause leaking. The pouch is difficult to change when full.

55. A. When the CNA recognizes that he or she may be becoming impatient with the resident, to prevent escalating the situation it is best for the CNA to leave the room and come back when he or she feels less impatient. Option B and D may escalate the situation. Option C will help the CNA, but it is not the first option.

56. B. The CNA should tell the nurse the resident's request, and he or she will evaluate and call the appropriate pastor. Option A is incorrect because the local church might not be the same denomination as the resident provided. Option C is incorrect because calling the doctor is not part of the CNA's scope of practice. Option D is incorrect because telling the resident that you are a pastor may make the resident uncomfortable and should be avoided.

57. C. The CNA should stop passive range of motion (PROM) when the resident complains of pain. Option A (stiffness) and B (weakness) are reasons for PROM to be performed. Use of passive range of motion increases flexibility and prevents stiffness. PROM is used for residents who are weak and may not be able to do active ROM. Option D is incorrect because PROM is not an exercise and will not increase muscle size.

58. D. Droplet precautions call for a mask to prevent transmission. Option A requires the use of gloves and possibly eye protection because there is a chance of splashing. Standard precautions (option B) is the term used for a set of infection control practices to prevent the transmission of diseases. Option C, contact precautions, require gloves and a gown.

59. A. A fracture is the cracking or breaking of bone. Option B is incorrect because a sprain is the twisting of ligaments. Option C is incorrect because a strain is the over-stretching or tearing of ligaments, and option D, laceration, is a disruption of skin.

60. B. When assisting a resident to ambulate, it is important for the CNA to continually ask if he or she has pain, is having any difficulty breathing, or if he or she is dizzy. Option A is incorrect because the CNA should stand beside the resident for safety if the resident begins to fall. Options C and D increase the likelihood of the resident or the CNA being distracted and introduces the possibility of falling or injury.

61. B. The CNA prevents spreading germs from one person to another by washing his or her hands when entering a room and leaving the room. Option A is correct when there is a possibility of respiratory contamination. Option C, bathing, can help to prevent infection by helping to keep the skin intact and moist. Option D does not prevent contamination.

62. C. The CNA is not to share the resident's information with anyone but the health-care worker who is taking care of him or her. The information provided in options A, B, and C is given to those who are responsible to help care for the resident.

63. B. The CNA should report the finding to the nurse and then follow through with applying lotion and gently massaging the area if directed by the nurse. If the resident is not changing positions often, the CNA will need to turn the resident more often, (D) but at least every 2 hours.

64. C. The resident has a right to religious beliefs and practices. The CNA should give the resident and his wife the privacy and time to pray. Options A, B, and D do not show the resident respect for his beliefs or privacy to practice those beliefs.

65. A. Kosher meals are prepared by special vendors who deliver kosher meals to the facility to be served to residents. Option B is incorrect because a kosher diet is a daily diet. Option C is incorrect because the meals have strict preparation requirements, and option D is incorrect because the rabbi does not prepare the meals.

66. B. A resident who is conscious needs to be sitting up (Fowler's position) when oral care is provided in order to prevent aspiration. Option A is used when the resident is unconscious; options C and D would risk the resident's aspirating while oral care is being provided.

67. C. The safest way to dress a resident is to begin with the weak side to lessen the risk of the resident's falling. Options A, B, and D would increase the risk of the resident's falling or not being able to complete the task.

68. A. Mild cognitive impairment is manifested by memory loss. As the impairment worsens, the resident will have trouble remembering how to dress (B), eat (C), and walk (D).

69. **B.** A barrier between the cold compress and skin is needed to prevent skin breakdown. Option A will increase the risk of skin damage. The cold pack should be left in place for only 20 minutes at time. Option C, putting on a heating pad after a cold pack, would decrease the effect of the cold pack. Option D should be performed only if the area is soiled.

70. **C.** Aspiration precautions include providing small amounts of food to the resident. Option A suggests the resident can be in any position to eat, but the resident should be in a high-Fowler's position to eat to prevent aspiration (B). The resident should be provided thickened liquids (A), not just liquids, and the resident should be provided oral care before and after eating (D), not at bedtime only.

71. **A.** The team member responsible for developing a discharge plan for a resident is the social worker. Option A is incorrect because the dietitian develops the resident's nutritional plan. Option C is incorrect because the CNA carries out the resident's plan of care. Option D is incorrect because the physical therapist assesses and develops plans to increases the resident's ROM and strength.

72. **D.** All the devices listed are examples of assistive devices. Canes, walkers, and wheelchairs assist the individual in mobility.

73. **C.** The goal of restorative care is to promote independence in activities of daily living. Options A and D will increase the resident's negative feelings about not being able to care for himself or herself and make him or her not want to continue in the process. Option B is incorrect because members of the team should encourage the resident in each small goal that is accomplished so that the resident knows that he or she is improving.

74. **A, B, C, and D.** The goals of restorative care include decreasing falls and injuries, promoting activity and mobility, and increasing muscle strength.

75. **D.** New residents may have difficulty adjusting to their loss of their independence, home, health, and belongings. The CNA can help by letting the resident make his or her own choices as much as possible, not make the choices for him or her. Encourage the resident to be involved and to get to know the other residents, rather than to stay isolated (B). Bringing personal items from home will make the resident feel more at home (C).

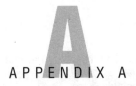

APPENDIX A

Nursing Assistant Test Cross-Reference

The tables in this appendix provide a cross-reference for the Practice Exam I, Practice Exam II, and Practice Exam III questions to the categories assigned in the Certified Nursing Assistant written exam (WE). Based on how well you do on the question type by category, this gives you a good idea of the categories in which you might need to study more rigorously.

TABLE A.1   Practice Exam I Question Cross-Reference by Category

Category	Number of Questions	Question Numbers
Activities of daily living	10	22, 29, 30, 35, 44, 45, 55, 61, 65, 73
Basic nursing skills	30	3, 6, 8, 10, 11, 13, 16, 23, 24, 33, 34, 40, 43, 47, 49, 50, 51, 52, 56, 60, 63, 64, 66, 67, 68, 70, 71, 72, 74, 75
Restorative skills	6	9, 12, 20, 26, 27, 38
Emotional and mental	8	2, 5, 31, 37, 57, 58, 59, 62
Spiritual and cultural issues	2	18, 25
Communication	6	7, 14, 19, 42, 48, 53
Client rights	5	28, 36, 39, 54, 69
Legal and ethical behavior	2	4, 21
Member of heath-care team	6	1, 15, 17, 32, 41, 46
TOTAL	75	

TABLE A.2   Practice Exam II Question Cross-Reference by Category

Category	Number of Questions	Question Numbers
Activities of daily living	10	7, 8, 18, 34, 41, 42, 43, 56, 63, 68
Basic nursing skills	30	1, 4, 5, 9, 10,13, 23, 24, 25, 28, 29, 30, 33, 36, 38, 39, 40, 46, 47, 48, 49, 52, 53, 55, 58, 60, 62, 66, 69, 75
Restorative skills	6	11, 15, 44, 45, 51, 72
Emotional and mental health needs	8	6, 35, 64, 65, 67, 70, 71, 74
Spiritual and cultural issues	2	2, 16
Communication	6	3, 14, 37, 50, 57, 59
Client rights	5	12, 22, 26, 27, 32
Legal and ethical behavior	2	20, 73
Member of heath care team	6	19, 21, 31, 54, 61, 56
TOTAL	75	

TABLE A.3   Practice Exam III Question Cross-Reference by Category

Category	Number of Questions	Question Numbers
Activities of daily living	10	7, 21, 23, 24, 35, 42, 66, 67, 70, 72
Client rights	5	9, 15, 18, 27, 28
Basic nursing skills	30	2, 4, 14, 20, 22, 25, 26, 30, 31, 32, 36, 37, 40, 41, 43, 44, 46, 47, 48, 49, 50, 51, 52, 54, 56, 58, 59, 61, 63, 69
Emotional and mental health needs	8	5, 8, 13, 19, 45, 62, 73, 75
Communication	6	11, 12, 33, 34, 53, 55,
Restorative skills	6	10, 57, 60, 68 ,71, 74
Spiritual and cultural issues	2	64, 65
Legal and ethical behavior	2	1, 3
Member of health-care team	6	6, 16, 17, 29, 38, 39
TOTAL	75	

Glossary

The definition of each term also lists the chapter in which the term first appears.

A

abduction   Movement of the limbs to the side, away from the middle of the body

abuse   Mistreatment

adduction   Movement of the limbs to the middle of the body

ADEs   Adverse drug effects

ADLs   Activities of daily living such as eating, bathing, grooming, walking, and toileting

advance directive   Legal and lay documents that specify certain aspects of care for individuals should they become unable to communicate their preferences

AIDS   Acquired Immunodeficiency Syndrome; late-stage infection by HIV

airborne transmission   Carried by air

Alzheimer's disease   Type of irreversible dementia in which cognitive function is progressively lost

a.m. care   Personal care provided in the morning hours to refresh; usually includes face and handwashing, tooth brushing, grooming, and toileting

ambulation   The act of walking

ambulation assistive device   Any device used to assist in walking such as a cane, crutches, or a walker

AMI Acute myocardial infarction; heart attack

analgesia Without pain; reduction of the sensation of pain

angina Chest pain

antisepsis The process of inhibiting growth of some microorganisms

aphasia Any speech deficit or loss of speech, writing, or signs, or loss of ability to comprehend spoken or written language due to disease or injury of the cerebral cortex

apical pulse The pulse heard at the apex (tip) of the heart

arteriosclerotic Narrowing and hardening of an artery

assault An attempt or threat to touch someone unjustifiably

atrophy Wasting away; decreased size of an organ or tissue

autonomy Being independent and self directed without outside control; able to make own decisions

axilla Armpit

B

bacteria Microorganisms

battery Willful or negligent touching of a person or personal belongings

beneficence Doing good for others

biohazardous waste Harmful or potentially harmful wastes

blood pressure The amount of pressure exerted against an artery when blood flows through it

blood-borne pathogens Microorganisms carried through the blood stream

body alignment Positioning the body in a straight line

body image How a person perceives his or her body

body mechanics Using the body safely and efficiently

body temperature The heat produced by the body

Braden scale A tool used to assess the degree to which a person is at risk for developing a pressure ulcer

C

calorie The amount of energy created by a nutrient or food

carbohydrates Food source; starches and sugars

cardiac arrest Condition in which the heart stops beating

caring characteristics Personal characteristics such as empathy and positive regard for others

cerebral vascular accident (CVA) A brain attack or stroke

Cheyne-Stokes respirations Breathing cycle of rapid breathing, followed by slow breathing and periods where breathing stops

chronic illness Illness that lasts for an extended period of time

coccyx Tailbone

code of ethics Formal written statement of beliefs of a group's ideals and values; a set of principles that reflects moral judgments and serves as standard for actions

colostomy   An artificial opening into the colon

comatose   Condition in which a person is unconscious

commode   A portable device used for toileting

communicable disease   A disease that can spread from one person to another

communication   The sharing of thoughts and ideas

competency   The knowledge and skill required to perform tasks correctly

confidentiality   Keeping information about someone private, telling only to other health team members as appropriate

congestive heart failure   Medical condition in which the heart fails to pump blood efficiently, causing fluid and blood to back up into the lungs or extremities

contact isolation   Methods used to decrease exposure to pathogens by direct contact of an infectious person or with contaminated objects in the environment

contagion   Pathogen that can be spread from one person or surface to another

continuing education   Formal learning activities that increase professional knowledge or skill

contracture   A permanent shortening of a muscle resulting in the shortening of associated tendons and ligaments

convalescence   The period of recovery from an illness or injury

coronary arteries   Arteries that supply the heart muscle with blood and oxygen

CPR   Cardiopulmonary resuscitation; methods to restore the heartbeat, circulation, and respirations

cultural diversity   Traditions, attitudes, and behaviors of persons who identify with a particular group or society

CVA   Cerebrovascular accident; stroke

cyanosis   Blue color of the skin due to lack of oxygen to the tissues

D

dangling   Sitting on the side of the bed with the feet hanging down

debilitated   Weakened or losing strength

defecate   To eliminate solid wastes from the body

dehydration   Lack of fluid in the body

delirium   Reversible, abrupt onset of confusion

delusion   False idea of reality

dementia   Cognitive impairment that is often progressive and permanent

dentition   The type and arrangement of teeth

dentures   Artificial teeth

diabetes   Endocrine disorder marked by inability of the pancreas to change carbohydrates into fuel needed for energy

diastolic pressure   The pressure exerted against the arterial walls when the ventricles are at rest

Director of Nursing (D.O.N)   Licensed nurse who has administrative responsibilities to supervise the nursing care of a facility

disoriented   Confused as to person, place, time, or circumstance

DNR   Do not resuscitate; order written by physician that prevents nursing staff from performing CPR or other life-saving measures

domestic violence   Harm committed on another family member

dorsiflexion   Bending a body part toward the posterior or the body

droplet transmission   Travel of droplet, or drop, through the expired air

dysphagia   Difficulty or inability to swallow

dyspnea   Difficult breathing

dysuria   Painful or difficult urination

E

ecchymosis   Bruise

edema   Swelling of tissues caused by accumulation of fluid

emaciated   Extremely thin; wasted

embolus   A substance (blood clot or air) that moves from its original location

emesis   Vomited material

empathy   The ability to communicate understanding of what another person is feeling or experiencing

end of life issues   Issues relating to death and dying

enema   A solution introduced into the rectum or colon to expel feces or flatus

enteral nutrition   Providing nutrition for someone unable to consume food normally; formula is introduced through a tube into the stomach of duodenum

ethics   Rules of principles governing right behavior

euthanasia   The deliberate ending of life of people with terminal illness or unbearable suffering

extension   Movement that brings the limb into or towards a straight position; opposite of flexion

F

false imprisonment   Unlawful restraint or detention of a person against his or her will

fecal impaction   Hard, retained feces that cannot be expelled

fever   Elevated body temperature

first aid   Immediate care given to an injured or acutely ill person before the arrival of the doctor or transportation to the hospital

flaccid   Limp

flatus   Gas in the digestive tract

flexion   Movement that brings the limb into or towards a bent position; opposite of extension

Fowler's position   Position of the body in semi-sitting upright position

fracture   Break

G

G tube   Gastric tube; placed directly into the stomach for feeding

gait-transfer belt   Cloth belt worn by the resident to assist with movement and ambulation

gatch handle   Handle at the foot of the bed used to change the bed's position

geri chair   Special chair that assists in positioning a resident to increase body alignment and comfort

geriatric   Medical care of older adults

gerontology   The study of aging and older adults

graduate   A round cylinder with markings to measure amount of liquid

grief process   Stages of emotional reactions to loss

gurney   A litter with wheels used to transport residents

H

hallucination   Falsely seeing, hearing, or smelling something that does not exist

hemiplegia   Paralysis or lack of sensation on one side of the body in the vertical plane

hemorrhage   Excessive bleeding

Hepatitis B virus (HBV)   Virus that attacks the liver

Hepatitis C virus (HCV)   Virus that attacks the liver; relies on HBV for transmission

holistic health care   Health care that considers the needs of the entire individual

from a physical, psychological, and spiritual perspective

hospice   Organization dedicated to end-of-life care for individuals and their caregivers and families

HS care   Care given to prepare the resident for sleep

human needs   Requirements to sustain health and happiness; air, food, safety and security, love and belonging, and self-actualization

hydration   The amount of fluid in the body

hygiene   Rules for health and cleanliness

hyperglycemia   Excessive amounts of glucose in the blood

hypertension   A condition of consistently elevated blood pressure above 140/90; high blood pressure

hypoglycemia   Abnormally low amounts of glucose in the blood

hypotension   Abnormally low blood pressure

hypoxia   Decreased amount of oxygen in the blood

I

immobilize   Make immovable

incontinence   Condition in which the resident cannot control urinary or fecal elimination

infection control   The process of minimizing the growth of infection

infusion-IV therapy   Method of delivering fluids and medications with the use of a needle or catheter inserted into the vein

intake and output (I & O) The total amount of foods and fluids ingested and eliminated from the body

intubation Insertion of a tube into the airway to deliver oxygen to the lungs

isolation Protecting an infected person from spreading disease-causing microorganisms to others

K

ketones Waste products from the chemical breakdown of fats

KS Kaposi's sarcoma; a rare form of cancer seen in AIDS patients

L

lateral position Side-lying position

legal-ethical practice The lawful and correct way to perform professional duties

Licensed Practical Nurse (LPN) A licensed nurse who works under the direction of a registered nurse (RN) to plan and provide nursing care

logroll To move the body while maintaining straight alignment

long-term care resident A client who lives in a health-care facility designed to provide rehabilitation and personal care for an extended period of time

M

malnutrition Insufficient nourishment for the body

mechanical lift Device to assist in lifting a resident who cannot move by oneself

mechanical ventilator Machine that delivers oxygen to the lungs

medical asepsis An environment free of pathogens

medical liability Legal accountability for performance of duties to others

metastasis Invasion of cancer cells in a site distant from the original site of invasion

microorganisms Any plant or animal that cannot be seen by the naked eye

MRSA (methicillin-resistant Staphylococcus aureus) Type of microorganism that is not easily killed by methicillin; an antibiotic

N

nares Openings into the nose

neglect State of being improperly cared for (physically, psychologically, or emotionally) that results in harm

negligence Failure to care for someone, which results in harm

nocturia Excessive urination during the night hours

non-malfeasance Doing no harm

Noncompliance Deliberately ignoring a plan of care

NPO Nothing by mouth

Nurse Practice Act Law regulating professional practice of licensed nurses

Nursing Assistant-Nurse's Aide Individual trained to provide personal care under the supervision of a licensed nurse

nutrient Substance in food that supplies the body with fuel for energy

O

OBRA   Omnibus Budget Reconciliation Act; Federal law that protects the quality of health care. The act addresses the safety, health, and well-being of patients as well as the quality of education and training for nursing assistants.

opportunistic disease   Disease contracted due to the body's weakened immune system

oral hygiene   Care of the mouth, teeth, and gums

orthopneic position   Sitting position that improves breathing in which the client leans over an overbed table with arms supported on pillows

OSHA   Occupational Safety and Health Administration; a federal regulatory agency concerned with the health and safety of employees

oxygen   A colorless, odorless gas that is necessary for life

P

palliative care   Care for clients whose disease does not respond to treatment; comfort care

paralysis   Lack of movement of a body part

paraplegia   Paralysis in the lower half of the body

pathogen   Disease-causing microorganism

Patient Self Determination Act (PSDA) Federal law giving individuals the right to make health-care decisions expressed through written advance directives and to be informed of his or her rights to accept or refuse health care

PCP (Pneumocystis Carinii Pneumonia)   A rare form of pneumonia contracted by individuals with depressed immune systems such as AIDS

perineal care (peri-care)   Cleansing and care of the genital and anal areas of the body

peristalsis   Wave-like muscular contractions in the tubular structures of the digestive system to move food

plantar flexion   The act of being a body part to decrease the angle between the bones forming a joint

plaque   A build-up of cholesterol in the arteries

PO   Per os (Latin); by mouth

polyuria   Excessive urination

postmortem care   Care of the body after death

postoperative   After surgery

PPE   Personal protective equipment such as gown, gloves, and mask or face shield; used to protect from contamination by pathogens

pressure ulcer   Sore or lesion on the skin caused by undue pressure to the body part directly beneath it

prone position   Lying on the abdomen, face downward or to the side

prosthesis   A device that replaces a body part

Q

quadriplegia   Paralysis of both arms and legs

quality assurance   A process of evaluating a facility's services by comparing them to accepted standards

R

radial pulse   Feeling the pulse (heartbeat) in the radial artery

range of motion (ROM)   The degree of movement possible in a joint

rapport   A relationship of mutual understanding between two people

reality orientation   Process of reminding a resident of who he or she is, where he or she is, the current date and time and current events

Registered Nurse (RN)   Person educated and licensed to assess, plan, diagnose, provide, and evaluate nursing care

rescue breathing   Providing emergency oxygen through own expired air for residents who are not breathing; artificial respiration

Resident's Bill of Rights   Document outlining the rights of residents living in a long-term care facility

respirations   Breathes, including inspiration and expiration

respiratory arrest   Condition in which a resident stops breathing

respite care   Care given to provide rest and emotional support to caregivers

restorative care   Care directed to restoring function to its highest level

restraint   Any device used to keep a resident from walking away from a location

risk management   A system or process to reduce danger to residents and staff

role   A set of expectations about how a person occupying a particular position in society acts

role reversal   A situation in which a resident's role is changed from an expected one to a different, often lesser one

rotation   Turning on an axis

S

scabies   A contagious skin infection caused by infestation by the itch mite

seizure   Sudden contractions of muscles caused by erratic brain activity; convulsion

self-actualization   Highest level of human needs; self-fulfillment

sensory overload   Overstimulation of the nervous system

sensory stimulation   Excitation of sensory nerves

sexual harassment   Unwelcomed advances or suggestions with sexual advances or innuendos

sexually transmitted disease/illness (STD/STI)   Disease transmitted through sexual contact

shingles   Rash caused by the herpes virus

shroud   Cloth used to cover the deceased body

Sim's position   Semi-prone, side-lying position with lowermost arm at the back, the body resting on the chest, and the uppermost leg flexed

sphygmomanometer   Blood pressure cuff

sputum   Mucus secreted from the lungs, bronchi, and trachea

standard precautions   Procedures used to protect against exposure to resident's blood or body fluids

sterile   Free from all microorganisms

Sterile Technique   Keeping sterile objects sterile or free of all microorganisms

stethoscope   Device to transmit sounds from the body to the examiner's ears

stoma   Artificially created opening from a body's cavity to the outside of the body

stool   Solid waste products expelled from the body; feces

suffocation   Depriving of air exchange

suicidal ideation   Thoughts of suicide that includes a plan, method, and time line

Sundowner's Syndrome   Condition in which confusion and agitation increases during evening hours

supination   Turning upward

syncopy   Fainting; losing consciousness

systolic pressure   Pressure of blood against the arteries when the ventricles contract

T

terminal illness   Illness in which recovery is not anticipated

thrombus   Blood clot

TIA   Transient ischemic attack; condition in which the brain cells are temporarily deprived of sufficient oxygen

TPN   Total parenteral nutrition; method of delivering nutrients through the vein to meet daily caloric needs

tracheostomy   Artificial opening into the trachea

Tuberculosis (TB)   Infectious disease in which a bacterium invades the body, affecting the lungs, brain, or bones

tympanic membrane   Membrane separating the outer from the middle ear that helps transmit sound into the middle ear

U

urinate   To expel liquid wastes from the body; to void

V

values   Set of principles or beliefs held strongly by a person

ventilate   To allow air into the lungs

virus   A pathogen that grows after invading a body cell

void   To expel liquid wastes from the body

VRE (vancomycin-resistant Enterococcus)   Bacterium that is resistant to the antibiotic vancomycin

Index

D

Q

R

S

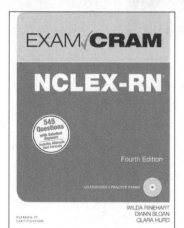

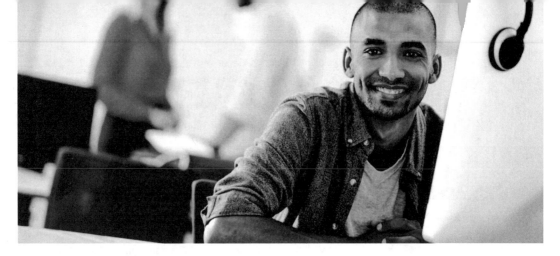